Understanding

HYSTERECTOMY
AND THE ALTERNATIVES

Dr Christine P. West

Published by Family Doctor Publications
in association with the British Medical Association

IMPORTANT

This book is intended not as a substitute for personal medical advice
but as a supplement to that advice for the patient who wishes to
understand more about his or her condition.

Before taking any form of treatment YOU SHOULD ALWAYS CONSULT
YOUR MEDICAL PRACTITIONER.

In particular (without limit) you should note that advances in medical
science occur rapidly and some of the information about drugs and
treatment contained in this booklet may very soon be out of date.

Family Doctor Publications, 10 Butchers Row, Banbury, Oxon OX16 8JH

Medical Editor: Dr Tony Smith
Consultant Editors: Chris McLaughlin
Cover Artist: Dave Eastbury
Medical Artist: Gillian Lee
Design: Fox Design, Godalming, Surrey
Printing: Reflex Litho, Thetford, Norfolk, using acid-free paper

ISBN: 1 898205 58 2

Contents

Introduction

Hysterectomy, which means the surgical removal of the uterus, is one of the most common operations performed in Western countries: by the age of 55, around one woman in five in Britain may expect to have lost her uterus. In some countries, such as the USA and Australia, this proportion is even higher, but it is lower in the Middle East because of cultural and religious differences. Fewer women have hysterectomies in Scandinavia where more use is made of drug treatment for menstrual disorders.

Around 10 years ago, an alternative operation was developed which may be a better option than hysterectomy for some women. In the new procedure, called endometrial ablation, only the lining of the uterus is removed and there is no surgical incision into the abdomen. This 'minimally invasive surgery' has advantages and drawbacks which will be explained in detail later in this booklet. Even with the new operation being used as an alternative, the numbers of hysterectomy operations being performed have continued to rise, but it remains to be seen whether this trend will continue.

Hysterectomy is different from other major operations because it often involves the removal of healthy, non-diseased organs. The table on page 2 gives the reasons why the operation is done: in over one-third of cases, there is some menstrual problem such as heavy bleeding for which no cause can be found. Medical treatments for most of these can be prescribed by your GP, but research has shown that some are more effective than others. In one recent year, over 800,000 prescriptions to relieve menstrual bleeding were written by GPs in England and Wales, while 73,000 women had hysterectomies and another 10,000 had endometrial ablations. These choices will be explained later in this booklet, but in general it can be said that hysterectomy is a very effective form of treatment and most women who have had the operation are satisfied with the results. Problems and regrets are most likely to arise if the operation has been done for the wrong reason or if the woman has uncertainties about it beforehand.

Not only will you, together with your doctor, have to make a choice between medical and surgical treatment and possibly between hysterectomy and endometrial ablation, but also, even if you decide to have a hysterectomy, you will be faced with more choices. In our mothers' day, hysterectomy almost certainly meant an abdominal operation, a 10-day stay in hospital and a prolonged convalescence. Nowadays, the uterus may be removed through the vagina with no abdominal scar. Sometimes, only part of the uterus is removed (subtotal hysterectomy).

WHO NEEDS A HYSTERECTOMY?

This list shows the most common reasons why a hysterectomy may be performed, although some of the conditions may also be treated without surgery.

Condition	Percentage
Fibroids	38.5
Menstrual problems	35.3
Prolapse	6.5
Cancer	5.6
Endometriosis	5.4
Other	8.7
TOTAL	100.0

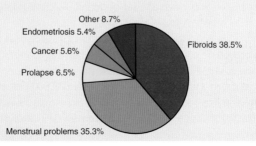

Other 8.7%
Endometriosis 5.4%
Cancer 5.6%
Prolapse 6.5%
Fibroids 38.5%
Menstrual problems 35.3%

Sometimes, the gynaecologist may recommend that the ovaries should be removed as well as the uterus. Again, all these alternatives will be fully explained in later chapters.

One more complicating factor is that your choice in terms of the type of surgery you have will depend on which hospital you go to, so that not all the options described in this booklet will be available to everyone. Some gynaecologists are involved in new developments; others prefer to use well-tried conventional methods until the newer ones have been more thoroughly assessed. Whether a hysterectomy is suggested may also depend on how familiar your GP is with the various medical treatments and on his or her attitude to hysterectomy.

How do you as the person most concerned fit into all this? Does it really matter what type of hysterectomy you have or where your scar is? Some women may feel that an early return to work is a disadvantage; for others there may be economic or professional reasons for wanting to minimise the recovery time. The object of this booklet is to explain the various treatment options available, both surgical and medical. It is designed to provide information that will supplement what you are told by your GP and gynaecologist, and the various health professionals whom you will meet. However, even as this booklet is being written, new developments are taking place and more information is being gathered about existing treatments. Thus, it can never be a substitute for first-hand information from your own hospital and informed discussion with the staff involved with your care.

KEY POINTS

✓ Hysterectomy is influenced by cultural attitudes and is more commonly carried out in some countries of the world (for example, the USA) than in others

✓ Over a third of hysterectomies involve the removal of a healthy uterus

✓ There are both medical and surgical alternatives to hysterectomy in most cases

✓ The decision to have a hysterectomy may involve more than one surgical option

The uterus: structure, function and common problems

The uterus, referred to since Biblical times as the 'womb', is a very remarkable organ, capable of expanding to contain a full-grown baby and of shedding its lining up to 500 times during your life at the time of your monthly period. The resultant

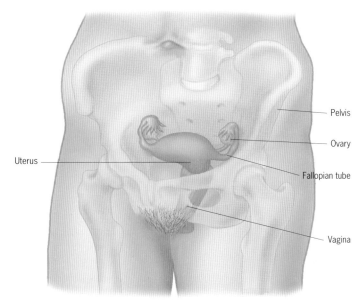

The uterus sits centrally in the pelvis, supported by strong fibrous structures called ligaments.

Pelvis

Ovary

Uterus

Fallopian tube

Vagina

stresses and strains on its supporting structures during pregnancies and the repeated shedding and re-growth of its lining may lead to problems such as prolapse or heavy menstrual bleeding. This chapter describes what the normal uterus and its related structures look like and how they work, and summarises what may go wrong.

When you're not pregnant, your uterus is approximately pear-sized. It has a thick muscular wall and a central cavity with a lining that is richly supplied with blood vessels. This lining is known as the endometrium and it provides nourishment for the embryo during the very early days of life. Otherwise, the lining of the uterus is shed each month, resulting in a flow of blood lasting for several days. This is known as the menstrual flow, menstruation or the monthly period. The uterine muscle wall expands greatly during pregnancy and strong contractions of this muscle wall during childbirth give rise to the pains of labour. You experience similar contractions on a much smaller scale during menstruation, and this is the cause of the period pain (dysmenorrhoea) which troubles so many women.

THE CERVIX

The cervix (or neck of the uterus) is the link between the uterus and the vagina (or birth canal) and is found at the top of the vagina. It is a firm, smooth, rounded structure with a central opening which:

- dilates (opens up) during labour

- allows menstrual blood to flow through it during your periods

- allows sperm to travel through it into your uterus during sexual intercourse.

When a doctor needs to look at your cervix, this can easily be done by inserting an instrument called a speculum into your vagina, and most women are used to having this done when their doctor performs routine smear tests.

THE FALLOPIAN TUBES AND OVARIES

The ovaries are situated on either side of the pelvis and are white, slightly knobbly and grape-sized. They are extremely important because they are the source of eggs and also of the hormones, oestrogen and progesterone (see below), which control the menstrual cycle. Each month an egg is released from one of the two ovaries in turn by a process called ovulation. This occurs at around day 14 of the menstrual cycle. The egg then enters the adjoining fallopian tube, one of two long, delicate structures attached to the uterus. This is

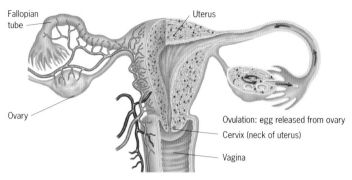

The ovaries are situated at either side of the uterus, connected to it by the fallopian tubes.

where the egg may meet up with sperm if you have had sexual intercourse, so beginning a pregnancy. A woman is born with a full supply of immature eggs and, from puberty onwards, these eggs gradually mature so that one is released each month until the egg supply finally runs out at the time of the menopause (see below).

SUPPORTING STRUCTURES

The uterus and cervix sit centrally in the pelvis, at the top of the vagina, supported by strong fibrous structures called ligaments. These ligaments are attached in turn to the bones of the pelvis. They are sufficiently elastic to allow them to stretch considerably during pregnancy and then return to their former size afterwards. In some women, particularly those who are past the menopause and those who have had children, this elasticity is reduced and the ligaments are weakened, leading to prolapse, or descent, of

the uterus and cervix. This causes discomfort, a dragging sensation and an awareness of a swelling or bulge at the vaginal opening.

In front of the vagina and close to the cervix is the bladder, which stores then gets rid of urine through a short narrow passageway called the urethra. Behind the vagina is the rectum (back passage) where the bowel expels faeces. These organs are supported by ligaments and muscles that stretch during pregnancy and childbirth. The ligaments and muscles that support the uterus, bladder and rectum, together with the walls of the vagina, are referred to as the 'pelvic floor'. When you're pregnant, you're taught how to exercise the muscles of your pelvic floor and improve their strength once you've had your baby. Women who have a pelvic operation will need to do the exercises too as they help to prevent any weakness developing and so keep the bowels and bladder working properly.

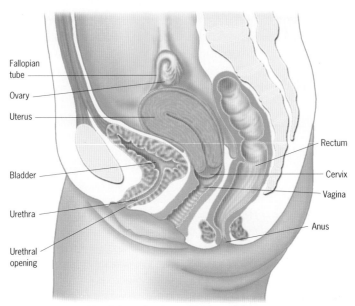

Female internal anatomy of the lower abdomen.

Fallopian tube

Ovary

Uterus

Bladder

Urethra

Urethral opening

Rectum

Cervix

Vagina

Anus

THE MENSTRUAL CYCLE

For around 40 years (on average, between the ages of 12 and 52), you experience monthly menstrual bleeding from the uterine lining, except for those times when you may be pregnant or breast-feeding. The average length of the menstrual cycle is 28 days but it is quite normal for it to vary between 24 and 35 days and occasionally longer. Some women find that the bleeding is accompanied or preceded by crampy pain (dysmenorrhoea or period pain), caused by uterine contractions. It may also be preceded by mood changes, bloating and breast tenderness, now referred to as the premenstrual syndrome

(PMS) and formerly called premenstrual tension (PMT). These symptoms are caused by the hormones produced in the ovaries, which act mainly on the uterus but also have effects elsewhere in the body. Different societies vary in their views about menstruation and, within all societies, individual women have vastly different experiences of their monthly periods. However, most look on menstruation as an unwelcome, albeit necessary, process.

FEMALE HORMONES

Oestrogen is the main female hormone produced by the ovaries and is responsible for the thickening of the uterine lining during the

HOW OESTROGEN AFFECTS THE BODY

Vagina	Moistens and lubricates Protects against infection
Breasts	Involved in breast development Causes activity in the glands of the breast (Causes cyclical swelling and discomfort in some women)
Bones	Important for bone development Protects against loss of bone mineral Helps to preserve bone strength
Other tissues	Keeps arterial walls healthy Protects against heart disease

menstrual cycle. It also affects the vagina, breasts, bones and other tissues (for example, walls of blood vessels).

Progesterone, the other female hormone, is produced only after the egg is released at ovulation and acts on the lining of the uterus, thickening it in preparation for a possible pregnancy. If you don't conceive that month, your hormone levels fall and your period starts.

The production of hormones and release of eggs from the ovaries are controlled by a small gland in the brain, called the pituitary gland, which regulates the length of the menstrual cycle.

THE MENOPAUSE

The menopause is the last menstrual period experienced by a woman. It occurs, at an average age of 52 in most Western countries. It happens when the supply of eggs in the ovaries eventually runs out. It may be sudden or gradual; some women experience increasing irregularity of their periods for months or even years in the lead-up to the menopause. As your supply of eggs declines, your hormone levels start to fall and this is what may cause the symptoms of hot flushes, night sweats, vaginal dryness and mood fluctuations that trouble many women. For most women, these symptoms are transient but a few find that they are a serious problem for quite a long time.

If this happens to you, your doctor may suggest treating the symptoms with hormone replacement therapy (HRT) and you may want to consider it even if the menopause doesn't affect you badly. This is because HRT may also have an important role in disease prevention: when your body stops producing the hormone oestrogen, you begin to lose calcium and minerals from your bones, and you also face an increased risk of developing heart disease. In addition, you may be predisposed to other health problems. These increased risks don't affect everyone after the menopause, but having your ovaries surgically removed at the time of hysterectomy is likely to aggravate these problems and this issue is discussed later in the book (see page 50).

COMMON DISORDERS OF THE UTERUS

Given the total number of menstrual cycles experienced by most women, it is not surprising that menstrual problems are common. These comprise painful periods, heavy periods, irregular bleeding and the premenstrual syndrome (PMS). Uterine fibroids are common benign tumours that may be a cause of heavy periods. Many women experience menstrual problems at some time in their lives but often these are temporary and settle down on their own or with simple treatment. Bleeding problems are particularly common in the lead-up to the menopause. Excessive bleeding is not only inconvenient, uncomfortable and embarrassing, it may also lead to anaemia (shortage of iron caused by blood loss).

Even after the menopause, the problems are not all over because this is the time when many women experience problems with prolapse of the uterus or vaginal walls. In particular, older women are more at risk of development of cancer of the uterine lining or ovaries, although fortunately these conditions are not common.

Hysterectomy is commonly recommended for menstrual problems and may be part of the treatment for many other gynaecological disorders. The most important of these are outlined below, and you will find more details on several of them in later chapters.

Heavy menstrual periods

Investigation may identify no serious cause for heavy periods and the problem is put down to a disorder of the shedding and re-growth of the uterine lining – so-called dysfunctional uterine bleeding. Menstruation is a very complex process and one that is not yet fully understood. It is likely that repeated menstrual cycles lead to disorders in this process because periods tend to get heavier as women get older. Another factor may be that some women become very intolerant of their periods once they have completed their families and are less prepared to put up with the monthly inconvenience. In some cases, the problem is related to changes in the levels of hormones produced by the ovaries in the lead-up to the menopause. More specifically, some women stop producing progesterone although their ovaries still release oestrogen. This means that there is not enough progesterone to counteract the build-up of the uterine lining which is caused by oestrogen. This leads to heavy, irregular or frequent bleeding.

In the absence of an obvious cause for the bleeding, decisions about treatment must depend largely on the severity of the symptoms, the impact they are having on the lifestyle and commitments of an individual woman, and whether heavy bleeding has led to anaemia. You should always be offered medical treatment in the first instance and it often works (see page 22). Endometrial ablation can also be helpful if you have dysfunctional uterine bleeding (see page 42).

If these measures fail, removal of the uterus, albeit rather drastic, will guarantee permanent relief but, as major surgery is involved, the risks as well as the benefits must always be fully considered (see page 58).

Uterine fibroids

Fibroids are rounded swellings of various sizes, composed of muscle and fibrous tissue, which grow in the wall of the uterus. They are extremely common and do not always cause symptoms, but, if they distort the cavity of the uterus, they may be a cause of heavy bleeding. Heavy periods caused by fibroids may be treated medically (see page 28), but this is less successful if the fibroids are numerous or large because medical treatments will not permanently shrink the fibroids. Similarly, endometrial ablation may not be possible or is less likely to succeed if there are large fibroids. Fibroids can be removed individually without removing the whole uterus (see page 47), but this type of operation, known as myomectomy, is usually offered only to women who may want to have children in future. However, if you have completed your family and are troubled by symptoms such as heavy bleeding or pelvic pressure, hysterectomy will bring a much welcomed relief.

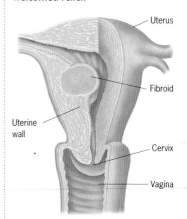

Uterine fibroids can grow in the wall of the uterus.

Menstrual pain

Only rarely is hysterectomy recommended for relief of menstrual pain because in most cases it responds to simple medical treatments, such as pain-killers or the oral contraceptive pill. Severe pain associated with menstruation, which is not relieved by standard medical treatments, may be caused by endometriosis (see below and page 27). Another condition, more common in older women who have had children, is 'pelvic congestion syndrome' in which periods are both painful and heavy with a build-up of pain, including backache and painful intercourse, in the lead-up to the period. Similar symptoms are caused by adenomyosis (see page 12) but this condition is difficult to diagnose. Hormonal therapies including the 'pill' can be successful by blocking ovulation and the hormone changes that follow because these may trigger pelvic pain in some women. Hormones can also be used to stop the menstrual cycle altogether. If this is not successful, hysterectomy is a possible option. Some women with symptoms of pelvic congestion have underlying problems such as stress or a depressive illness which may be aggravating the menstrual problem. It is important to appreciate that, if your pelvic pain is not related to the menstrual cycle, it is not likely to improve after a hysterectomy.

Severe or persistent endometriosis

Endometriosis arises because some women shed a little of the lining of their womb through their fallopian tubes in to the pelvis during menstruation. If this uterine lining tissue remains on the ligaments behind the uterus or on the ovaries, it may respond to the hormone changes of the menstrual cycle, giving rise to additional pain before or during menstruation. It may also cause deep discomfort or pain during intercourse. Even if endometriosis symptoms are improved with medical treatment (see page 27), the condition tends to recur and removal of the ovaries, together with hysterectomy, is a possible long-term solution.

In cases of severe endometriosis, there may be adhesions (scar tissue) in the pelvis, causing the uterus and ovaries to stick to other structures, such as the bowel and bladder, making a hysterectomy potentially difficult. When this happens, it is necessary to remove the ovaries as well because the condition is dependent on natural hormone production. Severe endometriosis may be a cause of infertility and this may make the decision to have a hysterectomy difficult for those women who are hoping to have one or more children in the future. In this situation, it is particularly important

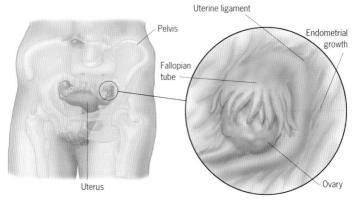

Endometriosis may cause the ovaries and uterus to stick to other structures, making hysterectomy potentially difficult.

that all alternative options are fully considered.

Although endometriosis is hormone dependent, most women can take HRT if they lose their ovaries. However, it may be necessary to give progesterone together with the oestrogen to prevent the oestrogen stimulating any remaining endometriotic tissue, if there is concern that the endometriosis has not been completely removed.

Adenomyosis

This condition causes heavy and painful periods as a result of the presence of uterine lining tissue in the uterine wall, causing the uterus to be tender and bulky. In contrast to endometriosis, which is more common in women who have not had children, adenomyosis usually occurs in women who have had several pregnancies. It

may develop as a complication of endometrial ablation. It can be treated medically but hysterectomy may be recommended if medical treatments are not successful. The diagnosis of adenomyosis is difficult to make on the basis of standard investigations because it is not visible on hysteroscopy or ultrasound scanning, and cannot be detected on an endometrial biopsy. Most cases are discovered only after a hysterectomy has been performed and the uterus examined by a pathologist.

Uterine prolapse

A uterine prolapse is the descent of the uterus and cervix so that they no longer sit up at the top of the vagina, but can be felt lower down, sometimes as far down as the vaginal opening. Prolapse of the uterus is caused by weakness of its supporting structures, usually as a consequence of child-bearing. You are most likely to develop it after rather than before the menopause and it is usually accompanied by prolapse of the vaginal walls. When it happens, you experience a dragging sensation and you and/or your doctor may feel a smooth swelling at the vaginal opening. Some women tolerate a prolapse for many years and come to no harm, but it can be a considerable nuisance and restrict your activities unnecessarily. If it is very large, the skin over the prolapse may become irritated by contact with underclothing, leading to discharge and even bleeding.

Minor degrees of prolapse may not require an operation or may be treated by a pelvic floor repair which leaves the uterus intact. However, removal of the uterus through the vagina (vaginal hysterectomy) together with repair of the pelvic floor is usually recommended if the prolapse is large. When a woman develops a prolapse before she has had all the children she would like, she will usually be advised to delay having surgical treatment until her family is complete. A ring pessary can be fitted as a temporary measure to support the pelvic floor. Ring pessaries are also suitable for the treatment of women who are not well enough to undergo an operation.

Ovarian cysts and tumours

An ovarian cyst is a collection of fluid within the ovary. Small cysts commonly develop as a complication of the menstrual cycle and normally do not require any treatment because they go away on their own. Larger cysts can be drained or removed without removing the ovary. If the ultrasound scan

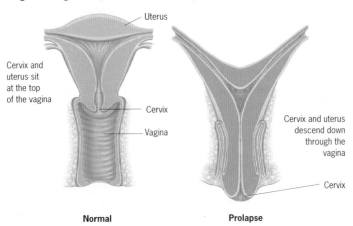

Cervix and uterus sit at the top of the vagina

Uterus

Cervix

Vagina

Cervix and uterus descend down through the vagina

Cervix

Normal

Prolapse

Uterine prolapse is the descent of the uterus and cervix through the vagina.

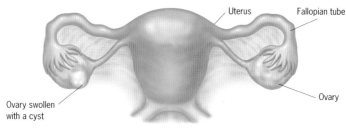

Uterus

Fallopian tube

Ovary

Ovary swollen
with a cyst

Ovarian cysts.

shows that the cyst is made up of solid areas as well as fluid, or if there is a solid swelling on the ovary (an ovarian tumour), it may be necessary to remove the whole ovary. If the cyst or tumour is very large or if there is doubt about its nature, your gynaecologist may recommend removal of the uterus and the other ovary, provided that you do not wish to have any more children. This is especially likely if there is concern that the cyst may be malignant (cancerous). Although most ovarian cysts are benign, there is a greater risk of cancerous changes if it is very large. Scans and blood tests are helpful in predicting whether an ovarian cyst is malignant. There is also a small risk that a similar cyst may develop at a later stage in the other ovary. More information is given about the treatment of ovarian cancer in a later chapter.

PREMENSTRUAL SYNDROME

Hysterectomy is sometimes recommended for women with severe premenstrual mood swings (premenstrual syndrome or PMS).

However, this is unlikely to help unless you also have significant problems with heavy bleeding or menstrual pain. Some women with very severe PMS benefit from removal of their ovaries, but this is a very drastic measure and does not guarantee a cure. Long-term treatment with hormone replacement therapy (HRT) is essential for women who lose their ovaries at a young age. As this is given continuously and at a low dose, it is unlikely to lead to a recurrence of the PMS symptoms, although some women with PMS are unusually sensitive to the effects of hormones and have difficulty with HRT (for more on medical treatments, see page 23).

WHO NEEDS A HYSTERECTOMY?

Most hysterectomies are done to relieve menstrual problems, particularly bleeding problems. Some of these will be the result of specific gynaecological disorders, most commonly fibroids. In many cases no specific cause can be found but simpler forms of therapy have failed to provide sufficient relief. Hysterectomy is rarely the only available solution for a menstrual problem but it is carried out with increasing frequency because of its success. Nevertheless, research has shown that the number of hysterectomies done for this reason varies greatly in different parts of the country and that this reflects differences of opinion among doctors. Thus the range of treatments you are offered may differ depending on where you live. In older women, most hysterectomies are done to treat uterine prolapse or as part of the treatment for certain forms of cancer. The subject of hysterectomy for cancer is discussed in the chapter starting on page 36.

KEY POINTS

✓ The menstrual cycle is controlled by the hormones oestrogen and progesterone, produced by the ovaries

✓ A woman sheds her uterine lining each month during menstruation – up to 500 times in her lifetime

✓ Common problems include heavy bleeding, menstrual pain, mood swings (PMS), fibroids, endometriosis and prolapse of the uterus

✓ Bleeding disorders are especially common near the menopause because of changes in hormone production by the ovaries

Examinations and tests

There are a number of ways in which menstrual problems can be investigated. These will depend on the nature of your problem and on your age at the time. You may not need any special investigations other than simple examination, particularly if you're under the age of 40, when serious underlying problems, such as cancer,

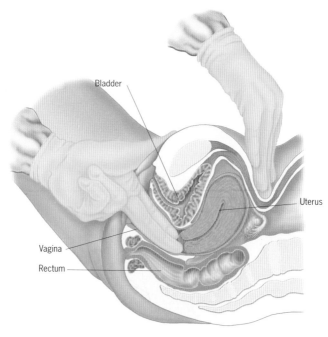

Bladder

Uterus

Vagina

Rectum

A simple pelvic (internal) examination.

are extremely rare. Often your doctor may prefer to try medical treatment to start with and only organise investigations if it doesn't work.

PELVIC (INTERNAL) EXAMINATION

A simple pelvic (internal) examination will enable your GP or gynaecologist to tell whether your uterus or ovaries are enlarged and whether there are any tender areas. He or she can inspect your cervix by inserting a plastic or metal instrument called a speculum into your vagina and a smear can be taken at the same time.

ULTRASOUND SCAN

An ultrasound scan will provide more information if your uterus or ovaries are felt to be enlarged, and detect any fibroids or ovarian cysts. This is a painless procedure which may be done externally by moving the scanning device over the skin of your lower abdomen or internally, via the vagina.

BLOOD TESTS

Blood tests are important in diagnosing anaemia, abnormalities of blood clotting and an overactive or underactive thyroid (which occasionally causes menstrual upset), and for measurement of hormone levels if you are thought to be nearing the menopause.

ENDOMETRIAL BIOPSY

Endometrial biopsy involves taking a sample of the lining of your uterus by first inserting a vaginal speculum and then passing a fine tube through your cervix. The sample is then sent to the laboratory for examination under the microscope. This may be necessary if you are

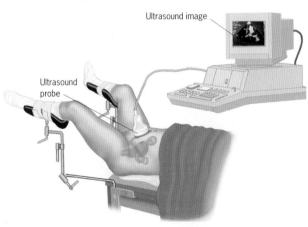

Ultrasound image

Ultrasound probe

An ultrasound investigation.

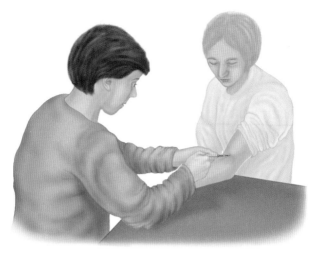

Blood test.

having irregular bleeding or additional bleeding in between periods. The biopsy can be taken in the clinic or surgery and takes only a couple of minutes, during which time you will experience mild discomfort, similar to a period pain.

HYSTEROSCOPY

Hysteroscopy is an examination of the inside of your uterus with an instrument (hysteroscope) which is fitted with a light source and camera so that a view of the uterine cavity can be seen on a screen.

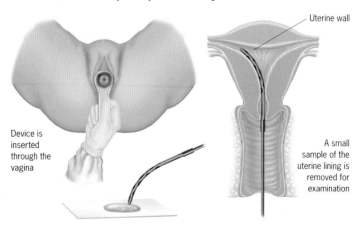

Uterine wall

Device is inserted through the vagina

A small sample of the uterine lining is removed for examination

Endometrial biopsy.

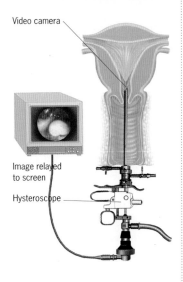

Hysteroscopy.

fibroids and is usually followed by an endometrial biopsy. In some hospitals hysteroscopy is done in the outpatient clinic; in others it is done as a day case procedure under a general anaesthetic.

The hysteroscope is passed through the cervix via the vagina, and gas or fluid is used to expand the cavity of your uterus. This technique can detect the presence of polyps and

DILATATION AND CURETTAGE

Dilatation and curettage (D&C) involves first stretching open the cervix (dilatation) and then scraping out the uterine lining (curettage). This has to be done under a general anaesthetic, and was the traditional method for investigating bleeding problems, but is now rarely used because the newer methods are more convenient and you don't normally need a general anaesthetic. However, they are not suitable for all women and some, particularly those with bleeding after the menopause, may still require a D&C. It

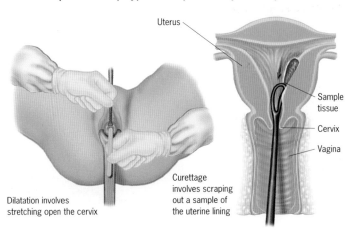

Dilatation involves stretching open the cervix

Curettage involves scraping out a sample of the uterine lining

Dilatation and curettage.

must be emphasised that a D&C has no value in the treatment of period problems, whatever you may have heard to the contrary.

DIAGNOSTIC LAPAROSCOPY

Diagnostic laparoscopy may be recommended if your problem is mainly one of abnormal pain associated with your periods. The external surface of the uterus as well as the fallopian tubes, ovaries and the surrounding structures are inspected through a laparoscope, linked up by a fibreoptic light source and a camera to a TV screen. Laparoscopy involves a general anaesthetic, one or two small abdominal incisions and a short stay in hospital, usually in a day surgery unit (no overnight stay).

One of the difficulties about treating women with heavy periods is that we have no accurate information about the amount of blood a woman is losing each month. Some hospitals measure menstrual blood loss by asking women to collect all their used pads and tampons. This is not a pleasant task but does provide invaluable information. For various reasons this is not done routinely and its use is normally confined to teaching hospitals undertaking research into menstrual problems. However, we do know from the results of such research that women tend to over-estimate the amount of blood that they are losing, and that more accurate information about actual blood loss may lead to fewer hysterectomies.

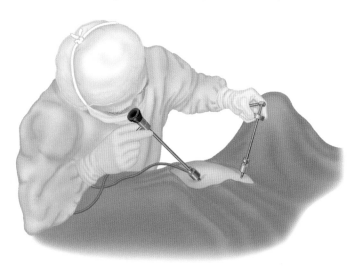

Diagnostic laparoscopy.

KEY POINTS

✓ Pelvic examination by a GP or gynaecologist allows detection of enlargement of the uterus or ovaries and the cervix can be inspected through a speculum

✓ Bleeding problems in women under 40 rarely have a serious cause and do not usually require investigation

✓ Investigations may involve blood tests, endometrial biopsy, ultrasound scan, hysteroscopy or laparoscopy

✓ A D&C does not help menstrual problems and is not usually needed for the investigation of abnormal bleeding

Drug treatments for menstrual problems

Menstrual problems are often temporary and may improve on their own or after a spell of medical treatment. Some such problems may be caused or aggravated by stress and improve when the cause of the stress is resolved. While your periods stop naturally at the time of the menopause, menstrual bleeding problems are particularly common in the lead-up to it – the so-called perimenopause. For women in this age group, it makes sense to persevere with medical treatments rather than to undergo surgery for which the benefit, in terms of days of bleeding prevented, may be relatively small.

Drug treatments for heavy or painful periods fall into two main categories: hormonal and non-hormonal. Although non-hormonal treatments are taken only during menstruation (to relieve immediate symptoms), hormonal preparations are taken for much longer in the cycle in order to achieve their effects. However, if bleeding is very irregular, hormonal therapies are more helpful because they can be used to regulate the bleeding pattern.

HEAVY AND PAINFUL PERIODS
Non-hormonal treatments
Non-hormonal preparations are used during the period itself to relieve symptoms: for example, pain-killers for menstrual cramps or headaches. Similarly there are medications that will help to reduce the amount of bleeding.

● **Mefenamic acid and related drugs:** Mefenamic acid (Ponstan) is the best known of a group of drugs that reduce both menstrual cramps and blood flow. This is available on prescription from your GP. They work by altering the production of substances called prostaglandins which play an important role in controlling menstruation. Their advantage is that they have minimal side effects. However, their effect on menstrual flow is only moderate, reducing blood loss by, on average, 30 per cent, which may be insufficient if your periods are very heavy.

If you are to gain any benefit, you have to start taking them just before the onset of bleeding and so timing may be difficult if your periods start without warning. This type of drug is most helpful for women with painful as well as

MEDICAL TREATMENTS FOR MENSTRUAL PROBLEMS

Generic name	Proprietary name	Comments
Non-hormonal treatment		
Mefenamic acid	Ponstan	Reduces menstrual bleeding and pain
Tranexamic acid	Cyclokapron	Reduction of blood loss only
Hormonal treatment		
Synthetic progesterones (progestogens)		
Norethisterone	Primolut N	Commonly prescribed for relief of irregular heavy bleeding
Medroxyprogesterone acetate	Provera	Commonly prescribed for treatment of endometriosis
Dydrogesterone	Duphaston	An alternative to the other progestogens
GnRH analogues		
Nafarelin	Synarel	Nasal spray (twice daily)
Buserelin	Suprefact	Nasal spray (three times daily)
Goserelin	Zoladex	Monthly injection
Leuprorelin acetate	Prostap SR	Monthly injection
Male hormone derivatives		
Danazol	Danol	Daily medication
Gestrinone	Dimetriose	Twice weekly medication

heavy periods and those with a regular cycle. Ibuprofen, which is available over the counter, belongs to the same group of drugs as mefenamic acid and is effective in relieving menstrual cramps, but its use for menstrual bleeding problems has not been fully tested. Drugs in this category may not be suitable for women prone to stomach upsets.

● **Tranexamic acid:** Tranexamic acid (Cyclokapron) acts on the mechanisms in the uterus for controlling bleeding during menstruation. It is available only on prescription from your GP. It reduces menstrual blood loss by an average of 50 per cent and is thus more effective than mefenamic acid, although it does not relieve menstrual cramps. It has the advantage that it is effective if you begin taking it once heavy bleeding has started, so you don't need to know exactly when that will happen. You can take it at the same time as a pain-killer if required. You need to take two tablets three or four times daily during the heavy days of the flow. Its use to treat heavy periods is relatively new in this country, but it has been used for many years with great success in Scandinavia where fewer women undergo hysterectomy. Side effects are few although it may cause gastric upsets. It is not recommended for women with a history of thrombosis.

Hormonal medications

● **The oral contraceptive pill:** The 'pill' or combined oral contraceptive pill (COCP) is an extremely effective treatment for the relief of both heavy and painful periods, because the combination of the hormones oestrogen and progesterone not only stops egg release, but also causes thinning of the uterine lining and reduces muscle wall cramps. It may also reduce symptoms of PMS. Unfortunately, many women mistrust the 'pill', partly because of bad publicity from the lay press which has tended to sensationalise reports of the risks while overlooking its many benefits. What is often not appreciated is that the 'pill' has other benefits besides those of contraception and relief of menstrual problems. Long-term users of the COCP have a significantly reduced risk of both uterine and ovarian cancer and are less likely to develop uterine fibroids.

Hormonally related side effects of the 'pill' are common and include bloating, breast tenderness, headaches and mood swings. These can sometimes be relieved by changing to a different brand. Serious side effects, although well publicised, are extremely rare. A minority of women are at greater risk of developing venous thrombosis (blood clots) if they take the 'pill'. Older women who smoke or who have high blood pressure are at more risk of heart disease, which is why it is not normally prescribed for women over the age of 35 who smoke. It is not suitable for women who are significantly overweight, have high blood pressure or a history of thrombosis. Although the 'pill' is most often prescribed for younger women, it can be used safely in women of all ages who are non-smokers and have no risk factors for heart or blood vessel disease.

● **Synthetic progesterone:** One of the most common causes of heavy, irregular bleeding is an alteration in the levels of hormones produced by the ovaries in the lead-up to the menopause. Provided that investigations are done to exclude a more serious cause, hormonal therapy is usually very effective in this situation. Irregular heavy bleeding may be caused by failure of the ovary to produce its second hormone, progesterone. Under the influence of oestrogen, the uterine lining continues to thicken and may haemorrhage. In these circumstances, bleeding can be controlled by taking synthetic progesterone, known as progestogen, to balance out the effect of the oestrogen. There are several forms of synthetic progesterone which can be taken in tablet form (see table on page 23). They are given in an initial course lasting 14 to 21 days to bring the bleeding

under control, and can then be prescribed for several months to regulate the cycle if it fails to settle down on its own. Some women experience side effects such as bloating, nausea and weight gain, but serious side effects are very rare. Natural progesterone is also available but has to be administered via the vagina because it is not absorbed through the stomach and high doses are required to control abnormal bleeding.

● **Hormone replacement therapy**: Hormone replacement therapy or HRT (oestrogen combined with progestogen) is sometimes used to treat bleeding irregularity in the lead-up to the menopause by regulating the cycle, although it may not reduce heavy bleeding if the cycle is regular. It is more effective in the control of irregular bleeding, particularly if there are symptoms such as hot flushes and night sweats which signify the approach of the menopause. Unlike the 'pill', it can be prescribed for smokers, regardless of age, and for many women with a history of heart disease, because HRT is composed of lower doses of natural hormones compared with the 'pill', which contains artificial hormones and at a higher dosage. However, any abnormal bleeding should first be investigated before HRT is prescribed.

Some women are concerned that taking HRT after their menopause may mean a return to the heavy bleeding they experienced previously. However, in practice, this may not be a problem as periods tend to be lighter with HRT. In the long term, many women on HRT can change to a bleed-free preparation in which both hormones are taken continuously, without a break, and the uterine lining eventually thins out. Irregular bleeding is common during the early weeks of this treatment but, if you are willing to persevere, the bleeding eventually stops altogether.

- **Progestogen-containing intrauterine system:** The progestogen-containing intrauterine system is a newer alternative suitable for women with heavy periods who favour a surgical solution but are anxious about the risks or about loss of fertility. There is one such system currently available, known as Mirena, but other similar systems are likely to be available in the future. It was originally developed as a contraceptive and this is currently its most important use. However, unlike older intrauterine contraceptive devices (coils), the Mirena was found to reduce menstrual bleeding dramatically – by over 90 per cent, as against 50 per cent for the 'pill' and with tranexamic acid.

Inserting the device into the uterus is simple and does not require an anaesthetic. Once in place, it remains in the uterine cavity where it releases a tiny amount of a progestogen (synthetic progesterone). This is sufficient to act on the uterine lining but negligible amounts are absorbed into the bloodstream so that hormonal effects elsewhere in the body are very minimal. The drawback is that, although heavy bleeding stops almost immediately, irregular light bleeding is very common in the first three to six months after insertion. Thus it may not appeal to you if you are seeking an instant cure.

Another advantage of the intrauterine system is that it relieves period cramps. The device is easy to remove and the effects are readily reversible, so it may suit you if you want to have more children in the future. However, it may not be suitable for women with large fibroids. The device is available in this country as a contraceptive, but at the time of writing is not yet officially licensed for the treatment of heavy periods. This means that it can be prescribed only by a hospital specialist. Once the licensing process is complete, a GP with the necessary experience will be able to prescribe and insert it, although some may prefer this to be done in hospital.

ENDOMETRIOSIS

If you experience severe pain during or before the onset of your period and/or find that sexual intercourse is painful, you may have a condition called endometriosis. The symptoms arise because uterine lining tissue (endometrium) has migrated from its proper place to the ligaments behind the uterus, on to the pelvic lining and/or the ovaries, and is stimulated to grow and shed each month by the hormones released by the ovaries.

It is diagnosed by laparoscopy (see page 20). There are several effective hormonal treatments which work by counteracting or suppressing the hormones released by the ovaries, leading to temporary cessation of the periods. Alternatively, small areas of endometriosis can be removed surgically (see page 48). These methods can relieve pain in the short term and often the condition improves on its own with time.

The problem is that endometriosis may recur once medical treatment is stopped and thus treatment may need to be repeated intermittently or continued long term. For some women, this may be preferable to surgical treatment, although hysterectomy may be the solution if the symptoms are severe or don't respond well enough to medical treatment (see page 11). Endometriosis is extremely variable in its extent, severity and duration, and it is difficult to generalise. Treatment should be tailored to the needs of the individual.

Some women find adequate relief of symptoms of endometriosis using non-hormonal treatments such as pain-killers. Alternative therapies (for example, homoeopathy, herbal preparations) have an important role for some women. As the symptoms of endometriosis are triggered by the hormones released by the ovaries, hormonal treatments are often prescribed to suppress this hormone production. Similarly, endometriosis is relieved by the natural menopause.

Simple hormone treatments

Used continuously, high doses of synthetic progesterone (progestogens) gradually shrink and inactivate deposits of endometriosis by counteracting the effects of oestrogen. They also suppress menstrual bleeding because of a similar thinning effect on the uterine lining. Progestogens have been used for many years in this way and their advantage over newer treatments (see below) is that they can be used for longer. However, side effects may occur, particularly irregular bleeding (spotting), bloating and fluid retention. An alternative is the combined oral contraceptive pill which works best for endometriosis if you take it continuously, without a monthly break.

- **GnRH analogues:** Gonadotrophin-releasing hormone (GnRH) analogues are relatively new drugs which are taken by nasal spray or by a monthly injection. They are synthetic versions of a natural hormone known as the gonadotrophin-releasing hormone and act via the pituitary gland to stop the ovaries producing hormones. This stops you having periods and deprives the areas of endometriosis of hormonal stimulation. They are very effective. The disadvantage is that, because your ovaries are no longer producing oestrogen, you may experience side effects such as hot flushes, night sweats and vaginal dryness. These are similar to the symptoms of the menopause. The other problem is that the GnRH analogues are not usually suitable for long-term use because lack of oestrogen may lead to loss of calcium and mineral from bones, leading to an increased future risk of osteoporosis. However, it is possible to take very low doses of oestrogen and progesterone in order to protect the bones if you need to remain on the treatment for a long time. This is an expensive form of treatment.

- **Male hormone derivatives:** Male hormone derivatives work by suppressing hormone release from the pituitary gland and the ovaries. Unlike the GnRH analogues, they do not cause bone loss or menopausal symptoms, but side effects of weight gain, fluid retention and greasy skin are very common. The best known of these drugs is danazol which you take in tablet form on a daily basis. A newer alternative is gestrinone which is more convenient in that you take it twice a week rather than every day. Side effects may include weight gain, fluid retention and greasy skin. There is also a small risk of growth of unwanted body hair and voice changes although fortunately these effects are rare. As a result, although they are very effective at relieving symptoms, they are usually used only in the short term.

UTERINE FIBROIDS

One of the most common causes of heavy bleeding is enlargement and distortion of the uterus by rounded outgrowths of the muscle wall called fibroids. These are benign (non-cancerous) tumours and vary in size, number and position. They are diagnosed by pelvic examination followed by an ultrasound scan. If they are very large they may cause pressure on the bowel or bladder; if small they may not cause any symptoms. Like endometriosis, uterine fibroids are dependent for their growth on normal ovarian hormone production and so tend to shrink naturally after the menopause. Treatments that lower hormone levels, such as GnRH analogues, make fibroids shrink in size, but they are less useful for this condition than they are for endometriosis because fibroids re-grow immediately the drug treatment is stopped. Other hormones such as synthetic progesterones, danazol and the oral contraceptive pill may be used to relieve blood loss resulting from fibroids, but do not cause shrinkage and are thus not helpful if the fibroids are large and causing pressure problems.

If you have smallish fibroids which are causing heavy periods, non-hormonal treatment with tranexamic acid may be very helpful and may cause fewer side effects than hormonal therapies. Bleeding resulting from fibroids may mean you develop anaemia, in which case a short course of an GnRH analogue may be prescribed to treat it, but you may ultimately need to have the fibroids removed surgically (see Myomectomy on page 47).

KEY POINTS

✓ Tranexamic acid (Cyclokapron) is a non-hormonal treatment that reduces bleeding

✓ The oral contraceptive pill relieves heavy bleeding and pain, and helps to protect against ovarian and uterine (endometrial) cancer

✓ Intrauterine devices that contain low doses of hormones are very effective in reducing heavy periods, but irregular bleeding is a problem initially

✓ Medical treatments are usually effective in the treatment of bleeding problems that occur in the lead-up to the menopause

✓ Medical treatments relieve the symptoms of fibroids and endometriosis but are not a long-term cure

Different types of hysterectomy

Once it has become clear that a hysterectomy is going to be the best form of treatment for your problems, you and your doctors may still need to decide which type of operation is best for you. It may mean removing all or part of your uterus and does not necessarily mean that your ovaries will be removed at the same time. If this is to be done, the reasons should be explained and discussed separately. This will be dealt with in detail in the next chapter.

ABDOMINAL HYSTERECTOMY

The uterus is removed through an abdominal incision, usually made low down, at or just above the top of the pubic hair line – the so-called 'bikini line'. If you have previously had an operation with a vertical scar (from just below the belly button to the hairline) this may be re-opened. If the uterus is very large

(for example, because you have large fibroids) or if there is a very large ovarian cyst, a vertical scar may be necessary. A vertical scar heals just as well as a bikini line scar, although it is more uncomfortable initially and is more visible and potentially slightly weaker in the long term because it cuts right through the centre of the muscle sheath that supports the abdominal

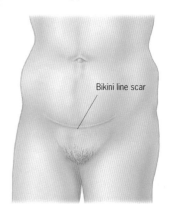

Bikini line scar

The uterus is removed at or just above the top of the pubic hair line – the 'bikini line'.

wall. Both types of abdominal incision involve going through the muscle layer as well as the skin and it takes time for this to heal and recover its strength afterwards.

Various methods are used to close the abdominal incision, including removable clips and staples, dissolving sutures (stitches that dissolve under the skin), and a single or a series of removable sutures. Healing occurs in the same way regardless of which method is used but, if you have encountered any problems with scars in the past and have any anxieties, it is important to let the hospital staff know.

In general, an abdominal hysterectomy involves a hospital stay of three to seven days and a recovery period varying between six and twelve weeks, depending on your general health, whether you develop any complications, your family commitments and what sort of job you do.

TOTAL ABDOMINAL HYSTERECTOMY

This is the most common operation and involves removal of the uterus and the cervix (neck of the womb), leaving a scar at the top of the vagina as well as the one on the abdomen. It does not necessarily include removal of the ovaries (see page 50). The advantage of removing the cervix is that it makes it

impossible for abnormal cellular changes to arise which might lead on to the development of cancer. Any such changes are detected when you have a cervical smear. Having a total hysterectomy means you'll never need another smear, providing that your cervix was entirely healthy and free of abnormal cellular changes when examined by the pathologist after the hysterectomy. Women who have had treatment for abnormal cells in the past, and those who aren't very good at going for smear checks or who want to avoid them in future should have the cervix as well as the uterus removed. On the other hand, if you have always had regular smears and they have always been negative, your chances of developing cervical cancer are very low and you may be suitable for a subtotal hysterectomy (see below).

SUBTOTAL ABDOMINAL HYSTERECTOMY

This involves removing the uterus but not the cervix and is a shorter, simpler and safer operation because the removal of the cervix tends to be the most difficult part. It may be recommended if the gynaecologist is concerned that removal of the cervix may be difficult (for example, if you have had a number of caesarean sections). The disadvantage is that you may still be at risk of abnormal cellular changes so you

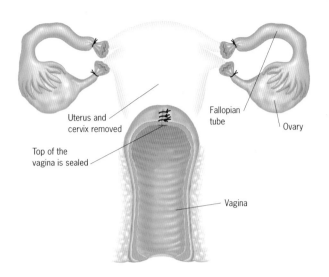

Total abdominal hysterectomy – removal of the uterus and cervix. In this illustration the ovaries have not been removed.

must continue to have regular cervical smears. Another potential problem is that leaving the cervix may also leave a fragment of the womb lining and some women experience continuing slight bleeding after subtotal hysterectomy. For some women stimulation of the cervix is important for sexual enjoyment and orgasm. However, research suggests that most women do not experience a deterioration in their sex lives after removal of the cervix. The views of gynaecologists differ regarding the pros and cons of total as compared with subtotal hysterectomy and this is partly because we do not actually know. Research is in progress which should provide us with an answer. In the

meantime some gynaecologists may offer you a choice; others may not.

VAGINAL HYSTERECTOMY

This is the method used for treatment of a prolapsed uterus. It can be combined with a pelvic floor repair if the walls of the vagina have prolapsed as well. Both the uterus and cervix are removed through an incision at the top of the vagina and so you aren't left with an abdominal scar. After an operation for prolapse, you'll be told to restrict certain activities, particularly those that involve lifting or straining, for the time being, to allow the pelvic floor to heal properly and to minimise the risk of a recurrence of the prolapse. You'll be given

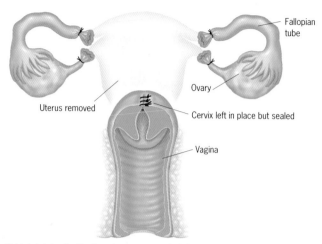

Fallopian tube

Ovary

Uterus removed

Cervix left in place but sealed

Vagina

Subtotal abdominal hysterectomy – removal of the uterus but not the cervix.
In this illustration the ovaries have not been removed.

advice about gradually returning to full activity by the physiotherapist who will also give you an exercise programme.

Until recently, women were rarely offered vaginal hysterectomy for relief of menstrual problems but this method has now become popular with many gynaecologists. This is partly because your hospital stay is shorter than with abdominal surgery, but also because postoperative discomfort is less and the recovery time is shorter than it is for abdominal hysterectomy. You can expect to be in hospital for two to four days and recovery is usually complete six to eight weeks after the operation.

If you're having your uterus removed because of menstrual problems, you may be offered vaginal hysterectomy, but this method is not suitable for everyone. It is very difficult to perform if there are large fibroids or an ovarian tumour. It is less likely to be offered to women who have had no children, those who have had previous pelvic operations or those who have had only caesarean section births. The gynaecologist who will be performing the surgery is the best judge of whether the operation can safely be carried out vaginally. When in doubt it is best to opt for an abdominal operation rather than run the risk of complications from a difficult vaginal operation. Currently only around 12 per cent of hysterectomies in this country are done vaginally, although this figure is very much higher in North America.

LAPAROSCOPICALLY ASSISTED HYSTERECTOMY

This uses methods that have become known as 'keyhole' surgery. Part of the operation is performed using a laparoscope and it is completed using conventional surgical methods, usually vaginal hysterectomy. The laparoscope is a viewing instrument which is inserted into the abdomen through a small incision below the umbilicus (belly button). It is connected to a camera and a fibreoptic cable, which allows the uterus and pelvis to be viewed on a screen. Two additional small incisions are made on either side of the abdomen for insertion of the instruments used to carry out the surgery.

Laparoscopically assisted hysterectomy is a relatively new procedure and not all gynaecologists have been trained to carry it out and not all hospitals have the special equipment required. In general, the operation takes longer to perform than the standard methods and there is a slightly greater risk of complications. The advantage is that there is a much smaller scar than for an abdominal hysterectomy and thus recovery should be quicker.

Usually the upper part of the uterus is divided from its supporting structures through the laparoscope and then the uterus and cervix are removed through the vagina (laparoscopically assisted vaginal hysterectomy). This makes it possible also to remove the ovaries if this is necessary. Some gynaecologists remove the uterus but not the cervix this way, but this technique is not widely available.

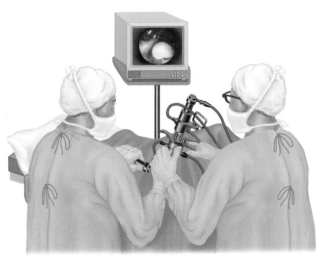

Laparoscopically assisted hysterectomy.

How the decision is made

This chapter has covered most of the methods used to remove a uterus but new ones are being devised all the time. In any case, your choices will depend on the facilities available in your particular area and also on the experience of the individual gynaecologist. All gynaecologists are currently trained to carry out abdominal hysterectomies and vaginal hysterectomies for prolapse safely, but many will be less willing to perform a vaginal hysterectomy for women who do not have a prolapse because the surgery is potentially more difficult. Only a minority of gynaecologists are currently trained to perform laparoscopically assisted hysterectomies and, if you are anxious to have this type of surgery, you may need to be referred to a specialist centre. At the end of the day, hysterectomy does guarantee relief of menstrual bleeding, no matter what method is used and no other treatment method will give this guarantee.

KEY POINTS

✓ A total hysterectomy involves removal of the uterus and cervix, but does not automatically include removal of the ovaries

✓ A subtotal hysterectomy preserves the cervix, but regular smears are still necessary afterwards

✓ Hysterectomies may be carried out abdominally, through the vagina or with the assistance of laparoscopy

✓ Recovery is quicker after a vaginal hysterectomy, but not all women are suitable for this type of operation

✓ Hysterectomy is the only treatment for menstrual problems that guarantees complete long-term relief of menstrual bleeding

Hysterectomy for cancer

Most hysterectomies are carried out to relieve problems that are troublesome or debilitating but not life threatening, so you are able to weigh up the pros and cons beforehand. When cancer of the uterus, cervix or ovaries is diagnosed, the decision about treatment usually has to be made very quickly in order to prevent the tumour spreading, and there may be no alternative to a hysterectomy. Nevertheless, it is still important that you fully understand the proposed treatment, whether you have any choices and what will happen afterwards. Ask a relative or friend to come to the hospital with you to help you remember what is said and write down what questions you want to ask.

Hysterectomy may be only one part of your treatment and several specialists are likely to be involved in deciding the best course of action, including the gynaecologist, a pathologist who is responsible for examining tissue specimens and an oncologist (cancer specialist) who will advise about the necessity for additional treatment, such as radiotherapy or chemotherapy. There are often specialised nurses attached to such a team and they can be a great help in providing explanations, reassurance and support.

CANCER OF THE ENDOMETRIUM (UTERINE LINING)

Endometrial cancer causes abnormal bleeding after the menopause or irregular bleeding in younger women. It is more common after the menopause and is extremely rare in women under the age of 40. The diagnosis is made by a pathologist following an examination of a sample from the uterine lining (endometrial biopsy – see page 17).

The endometrial lining is surrounded by the thick muscle wall of the uterus so it is rare for this type of cancer to spread beyond the uterus, and a hysterectomy therefore gives a very good chance of a complete cure. Your ovaries will also be removed because the cancer may spread from the uterus to the ovaries or abnormal hormone production by the ovaries may have been a cause of the cancer. If the pathologist who examines the uterus and ovaries after the operation has the slightest suspicion that the cancer may have spread beyond the uterus, a course of radiotherapy (X-ray therapy) will be recommended to destroy any cancer cells that may have entered the surrounding tissues with the object of achieving a complete cure.

The hysterectomy is normally performed through an abdominal incision, although occasionally the gynaecologist may decide that a vaginal or laparoscopically assisted approach is appropriate. Whatever method is used, it is likely that it will take a little longer than usual to recover fully afterwards, because the women concerned tend to be older than those having hysterectomies for other reasons.

As most women with cancer of the endometrium are already menopausal or beyond their fertile years, the decision to perform a hysterectomy is rarely a difficult one for the woman herself although there will always be exceptions to this, particularly for women who have never had children. Unfortunately, this form of cancer is more common in childless women. As cancer of the endometrium may be caused by high oestrogen levels, oestrogen-containing HRT cannot usually be prescribed. This may be a problem for premenopausal women if they develop troublesome menopausal symptoms after removal of their ovaries. You may be able to take preparations containing progesterone instead, but you will need to discuss this with your gynaecologist or oncologist.

CANCER OF THE CERVIX

This form of cancer affects the neck of the uterus and is usually prevented from developing by early detection of abnormal cells through the cervical smear programme. If your smear test shows up precancerous cells, they are removed by a procedure called colposcopy, which involves a detailed inspection of the cervix through a magnifying system (colposcope). This enables the removal of abnormal cells by simple treatments which leave the uterus and cervix to function normally. This pre-cancerous condition is known as cervical intraepithelial neoplasia (CIN) and must not be confused with cervical cancer itself.

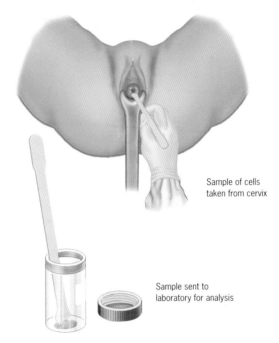

Sample of cells taken from cervix

Sample sent to laboratory for analysis

A cervical smear can enable the early detection of abnormal cells in the cervix.

Despite the effectiveness of the smear programme, some women still develop cervical cancer, sometimes at a relatively young age, before a woman has completed her family. If the tumour is fairly small, it can be treated by hysterectomy but, if it has started to spread, it cannot all be removed by hysterectomy and radiotherapy will be necessary, either as well as or instead of hysterectomy. Both these forms of treatment will result in loss of fertility, although a hysterectomy for cervical cancer does not usually involve removal of the ovaries. Theoretically, a woman who has a hysterectomy but still has her ovaries could have a child with a partner, but only with the use of in vitro fertilisation (IVF) and with the help of another woman willing to carry that child for them (a surrogate mother). Radiotherapy stops the ovaries from functioning so there is no prospect of future fertility. However, methods of retrieving and storing portions of ovarian tissue are currently being researched and may become available in the future. Therefore, any young woman with cervical cancer faced with loss of fertility should have the opportunity of discussing the implications and any available options before treatment is started.

A hysterectomy for cervical cancer is a very major operation because it involves removal of additional tissues besides and below the cervix, and also removal of the lymph nodes in the pelvis to which cancer may spread. In particular the bladder and bowels may take longer to return to normal. Loss of the ovaries or of their function after treatment of cervical cancer can be compensated for with HRT because this form of cancer is not influenced by hormones.

OVARIAN CANCER

This condition is less clear than the others described above because there are many different types of ovarian cancer and it is not always possible to diagnose its extent or even its presence in advance of an operation. A woman may therefore face uncertainties about the precise nature of an operation to remove the cancer until after it is over. Nevertheless, a woman's desire to retain her fertility will always be taken into consideration and is likely to influence decisions about her treatment.

The symptoms of ovarian cancer are very vague and varied, usually abdominal discomfort or swelling, possibly vague ill-health and weight loss. It may come to light because the woman herself or her doctor has

felt a swelling in her abdomen. The suspicion is then confirmed by the results of an ultrasound scan if one or both ovaries are seen to be very enlarged and suspicious in appearance. Blood tests may give additional information and sometimes a more detailed type of scan (computed tomography [CT] or magnetic resonance imaging [MRI] scan) is performed. Sometimes it is possible to be fairly confident about the diagnosis of cancer, but often there is uncertainty which can be resolved only by removal of the ovary and having it examined by the pathologist.

If a woman with suspected ovarian cancer has completed her family and/or is postmenopausal, she will most probably be advised to have both ovaries and the uterus removed in order to avoid the need for a second operation and to minimise the risk that the disease may come back. Even a benign tumour may develop in the other ovary in the future. If there are visible signs that the cancer has spread beyond the ovary, these areas are removed as well.

Ovarian cancer more commonly affects older women and is fortunately rare in women under 40. Its treatment in younger women always involves weighing up the risks of spread of the cancer against the risk that fertility will be lost, and the wishes and opinions of the woman

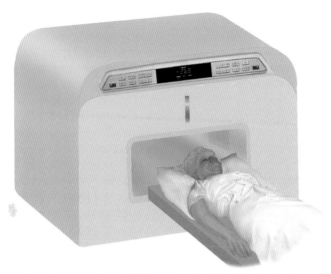

Magnetic resonance imaging (MRI) may sometimes be used to visualise the ovaries.

herself are always taken into consideration. It may be possible to remove only the affected ovary and leave the uterus and remaining ovary if the woman is anxious to retain her fertility, unless there is obvious spread of the tumour. Treatment of ovarian cancer in young women will usually involve chemotherapy (use of drugs that destroy cancer cells) and there is a risk that this may also damage the egg-producing cells in the remaining ovary, although it is usually possible to select drugs that minimise this risk.

FURTHER TREATMENT

Hysterectomy for cancer may be followed by additional treatment with radiotherapy or chemotherapy, depending on what is found during the operation and the results of the pathologist's tests on the tissues. As mentioned above, recommendations regarding further treatment are made by a team of specialists. Even if additional treatment is not required, further visits to the hospital will be necessary in order to check for any signs that the cancer may be recurring.

KEY POINTS

✓ Hysterectomy may be only one part of the treatment of cancer, together with chemotherapy and/or radiotherapy

✓ Most cancers of the uterus or ovaries occur in older women, beyond the age of the menopause

✓ In younger women, there should be full discussion of issues and options relating to fertility before treatment is commenced

✓ HRT is suitable for women after treatment of ovarian or cervical cancer, but not after treatment of uterine body (endometrial) cancer

Surgical alternatives to hysterectomy

Although surveys show that women are generally very satisfied with the results of a hysterectomy, there is concern that many women may be undergoing the operation even though they don't have any significant or serious disease within the uterus. In recent years surgical procedures have been developed in which the endometrium (the uterine lining) is removed or destroyed, leaving the remainder of the uterus and the ovaries undisturbed. This is known as endometrial ablation. This chapter also describes alternative surgical methods of treatment for endometriosis and uterine fibroids.

ENDOMETRIAL ABLATION

There are several ways in which this can be performed and they all avoid the need for a surgical incision. The methods used vary in cost and complexity, and whether they will be on offer in your hospital will depend on the preferences of local gynaecologists. Indeed, although some are very positive and enthusiastic about endometrial ablation, others continue to view it with scepticism so that in some hospitals it is not available at all. Most endometrial ablations are carried out under a general anaesthetic although, in some hospitals, it is available under a local anaesthetic. All procedures are carried out via the vagina, by passage of instruments into the cavity of the uterus through the cervix.

Endometrial resection

Endometrial resection and TCRE (transcervical resection of the endometrium) are terms used to describe the removal of the uterine lining in strips using a fine wire loop through which an electric current is passed (electrodiathermy). This heats up

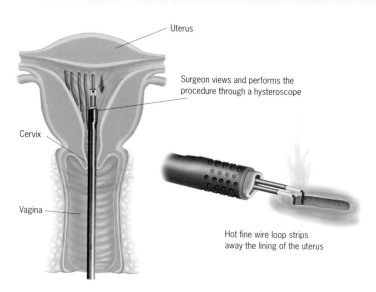

Uterus

Surgeon views and performs the procedure through a hysteroscope

Cervix

Vagina

Hot fine wire loop strips away the lining of the uterus

Endometrial resection.

and coagulates the muscle wall of the uterus at the same time as it strips away the lining, thus reducing the risk of haemorrhage. The wire loop is inserted down the side channel of an instrument called a hysteroscope so that the surgeon can watch the procedure on a screen. The uterine cavity is continuously flushed through with fluid to open it up and give a good view while simultaneously washing out blood and tissue debris and cooling the uterus down.

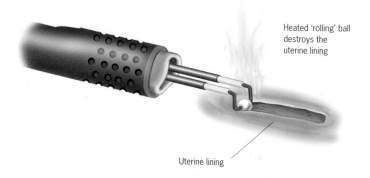

Heated 'rolling' ball destroys the uterine lining

Uterine lining

Roller ball endometrial ablation.

Roller ball endometrial ablation

This is similar to endometrial resection in that it uses heat generated by electricity (electrodiathermy) but the difference is that the uterine lining is destroyed by contact with the ball which is rolled slowly over the surface. Like endometrial resection, the procedure is done using a hysteroscope with constant fluid irrigation.

Laser endometrial ablation

This destroys the endometrium using heat generated by a laser. The laser beam is passed down the side arm of a hysteroscope and guided by the surgeon over the uterine lining. The laser is in many ways ideal for this task but has the disadvantage of being very expensive and beyond the price range of most NHS hospitals.

Radiofrequency ablation

This differs from the procedures described above in that it does not involve a hysteroscope or fluid irrigation. A probe of suitable size is inserted into the cavity of the uterus and a set amount of heat is applied for a specific length of time so as to destroy the endometrium. This technique is less commonly used than electrodiathermy methods because of the high cost of the equipment involved.

Uterine balloon therapy

This involves the insertion of a small balloon into the cavity of the uterus. This is filled with fluid so that it fits the shape of the cavity exactly. It is then heated to a temperature sufficient to destroy the endometrium. Although relatively new, it seems to work as well as other methods and is potentially safer; again it is quite costly to the NHS.

Other methods

Other methods are being developed all the time. You may read about one of these in a newspaper

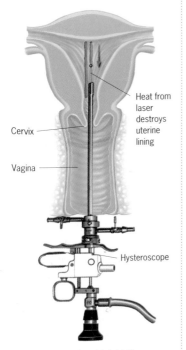

Laser endometrial ablation.

Cervix

Vagina

Heat from laser destroys uterine lining

Hysteroscope

or magazine, or even on the Internet, only to find that it is not available locally. This is because new treatments have to be thoroughly tested and compared with existing methods before they can be introduced more widely. Some hospitals will prefer existing methods; others may be involved in testing out one of the newer methods.

Drug treatment before endometrial ablation

During the menstrual cycle, the uterine lining gradually grows and thickens in preparation for possible pregnancy as described on page 8. It is very difficult to ablate or remove a thick endometrium and drugs are prescribed that thin the lining in preparation for surgery. These drugs – usually a GnRH analogue or danazol – are prescribed for around four weeks before surgery (see page 28). They are not usually required before radiofrequency ablation or uterine balloon therapy.

The advantages of endometrial ablation

Although most endometrial ablation operations are carried out under general, rather than local, anaesthetic, they can be performed on a day case basis or with, at most, an overnight hospital stay and recovery is considerably faster than after a hysterectomy. You will be able to take up your normal domestic activities after an average of two weeks and go back to work after three weeks – less than half the recovery time needed after a hysterectomy.

Possible complications

Although the principle behind these procedures is very simple and most take place uneventfully, there is a small risk of serious complications. As with all operations these include difficulties resulting from the use of the anaesthetic, excessive bleeding (haemorrhage) and infection. These complications are less likely following all methods of endometrial ablation than they are after a hysterectomy. However, there are complications that arise only after endometrial ablation. One is absorption into the circulation of the fluid used to flush out the uterine cavity. Absorption of small amounts is not a problem but if this is excessive it can put a strain on the heart and circulation – a condition known as fluid overload. Another possible and serious complication is perforation of the uterine wall by the instrument used to ablate or remove the uterine lining. If this isn't spotted immediately, it can result in damage to nearby structures, including the intestines and large blood vessels, and emergency surgery to repair the damage is then required.

Methods such as radiofrequency ablation and the hot balloon are in theory safer because they do not require the use of fluid irrigation; they are also less dependent on the skill and experience of the operator. Nevertheless, technical complications with the equipment have occurred and no method is entirely risk-free. Results of recent surveys have shown that between two and six per cent of endometrial ablation operations have serious complications and that the risk of complications is slightly higher with endometrial resection than with other methods.

How successful is endometrial ablation?

In the short term, endometrial ablation has many advantages over hysterectomy but, unlike hysterectomy, it does not guarantee to stop all menstrual bleeding in the future. Survey results indicate that, two to three years after the operation, around 20 per cent of women have no menstrual bleeding and 50 to 60 per cent have reduced bleeding, but up to 25 per cent find that there is no improvement or an actual worsening. The success rate declines with time and this is thought to be because the uterine lining gradually re-grows. The other problem is that results vary considerably, depending on the skill and experience of those carrying out the operations.

This situation is different with hysterectomy because, although short-term complication rates may differ between individual surgeons, overall success in terms of relief of bleeding problems is no different.

Although recent surveys suggest that up to three-quarters of the women treated with endometrial ablation are satisfied with the results – a higher proportion than for medical treatments – the fact remains that this has not resulted in fewer hysterectomies being carried out in the country as a whole.

Is endometrial ablation right for you?

If you have completed your family and are seeking relief of heavy bleeding, do not suffer much menstrual discomfort and wish to avoid major surgery, endometrial ablation is an option well worth considering. However, you should always try medical treatments first (see page 23).

This form of treatment is not suitable for women who may want to have children in the future. The procedure reduces fertility and, although some women have become pregnant after endometrial ablation, there is a significant risk of complications.

- Very painful periods are not likely to be relieved after endometrial ablation.

- Irregular bleeding may not improve after endometrial resection.

- This type of treatment is not recommended for women with a uterus enlarged by fibroids (see below).

If you want to stop having periods altogether rather than simply to reduce the monthly flow, you are likely to be disappointed by the results of endometrial ablation.

UTERINE FIBROIDS

In some instances, you may be offered an operation to treat fibroids which does not involve removing the uterus itself, but this will not be appropriate for everyone.

Myomectomy

Fibroids are one of the most common causes of heavy periods and one of the most common reasons why hysterectomy may be recommended. If you have not had children or want to have more in the future, it may be possible to remove the fibroids and preserve the uterus – an operation known as myomectomy. This is not easy to do from the surgeon's point of view, particularly if there are several fibroids, and in some cases they may be very numerous. It is normally done by open surgery unless the fibroids are within the uterine

cavity (see below). Laparoscopic (keyhole) methods may be used in some very specialised centres.

An operation to remove large fibroids may be complicated by heavy bleeding, so that a hysterectomy does have to be done, but this is fortunately rare. After a myomectomy, there is no guarantee that you can still become pregnant or that heavy bleeding will be cured and there is still a chance that further fibroids will grow in the future.

Is myomectomy right for you?

For the reasons outlined above, it does not make sense to opt for a myomectomy rather than a hysterectomy unless you are anxious to retain your uterus so that you can have children at some time in the future. However, if you have strong objections to hysterectomy for personal or cultural reasons, most gynaecologists will be sympathetic, provided that you fully understand the risks and limitations. An operation to remove fibroids should be done only if the fibroids are causing symptoms such as pressure or heavy bleeding, not just because they're there. Rarely, fibroids may be a cause of recurrent miscarriages, in which case they should be removed. However, most women with fibroids who conceive go on to have successful pregnancies. Similarly fibroids do not usually cause infertility although they are more common in women who have not had children.

Hysteroscopic myomectomy

Some women have fibroids that are situated within the uterine cavity, so-called submucous fibroids. If so, it may be possible to remove them with the aid of a hysteroscope, using methods similar to those described above. However, it is best for such procedures to be carried out in a hospital that specialises in hysteroscopic surgery because removal of fibroids in this way is difficult and requires considerable experience.

Fibroid embolisation

This is a new treatment that does not involve a surgical scar or a general anaesthetic. It involves the use of X-rays, which show up the blood supply to the uterus by dye injected through a very fine plastic tube inserted into the groin. Once the arteries (blood vessels) supplying the fibroids have been located, a special material is injected that blocks off (embolises) the blood supply. Initially, this causes as much pain as an operation and it is necessary to stay in hospital for one or two days. Embolisation results in shrinkage of the fibroids, but they do not disappear altogether. Results are still preliminary and the long-term success of the treatment is not

known, although it seems to relieve heavy bleeding and pressure symptoms in the short term. This form of treatment is not available in all hospitals and is still undergoing evaluation. It is not currently recommended for women planning to have children.

ENDOMETRIOSIS

Although a hysterectomy may sometimes be done to treat this condition (see page 11), alternative surgical techniques may sometimes be suitable. The diagnosis of endometriosis is usually made by laparoscopy (see page 20) and some gynaecologists will offer to treat small areas of endometriosis while they're doing the diagnostic laparoscopy operation. This can be done using electrodiathermy (direct heat generated by electrical energy), by laser or by other similar methods. If the endometriosis is more extensive, a second operation may be required to carry out this treatment, possibly after a course of drug treatment. Endometriosis that has resulted in the formation of ovarian cysts containing altered blood (endometriomas or chocolate cysts) requires surgical treatment, and this is often best done by laparoscopy rather than by open surgery, unless the cysts are very large.

The disadvantage of surgical as opposed to medical treatment to relieve the symptoms of endometriosis is that not all areas of endometriosis are visible and thus the surgery may not relieve the discomfort altogether. Often a combination of medical and surgical treatment is the most effective.

For women with severe endometriosis who want children, in vitro fertilisation (IVF) may be the best option and this can be combined with spells of medical treatment to relieve symptoms in between cycles of IVF.

Symptoms of endometriosis clear up during pregnancy and may be considerably improved thereafter, although a successful pregnancy does not guarantee a long-term cure of endometriosis.

KEY POINTS

✓ Endometrial ablation (removal or destruction of the uterine lining) is helpful in up to 70 per cent of women with heavy periods, but rarely stops bleeding altogether

✓ Endometrial ablation is not suitable for women who have not completed their families and may not relieve pelvic pain

✓ Endometriosis can be treated surgically without removal of the uterus or ovaries, but symptom relief may be only temporary

✓ Myomectomy is an operation to remove fibroids that preserves the uterus in women who hope to have children

✓ Embolisation is a new treatment of fibroids, but its long-term effectiveness is not yet known

Hysterectomy and your ovaries

Removal of the ovaries is not an automatic part of most hysterectomies, although it can be done at the same time and through the same surgical incision (scar). This should never be seen as a matter of convenience, because you are having an operation done anyway. The question of whether your ovaries should be removed is very important and must be given very careful and separate consideration. There will be some situations – for example, the treatment of endometriosis or certain forms of cancer – where removal of the ovaries is an important part of the treatment of the underlying problem. This does not apply to most hysterectomies carried out for the relief of menstrual problems.

WHAT YOUR OVARIES DO

The main function of your ovaries is the monthly release of eggs to enable you to conceive a baby. The

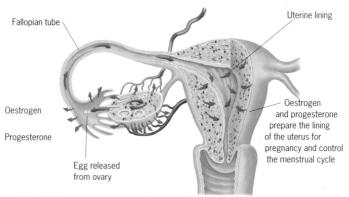

Fallopian tube

Uterine lining

Oestrogen

Progesterone

Oestrogen and progesterone prepare the lining of the uterus for pregnancy and control the menstrual cycle

Egg released from ovary

The main function of your ovaries is the monthly release of eggs to enable you to conceive a baby.

ovaries also produce the two hormones, oestrogen and progesterone, which prepare the lining of the uterus for pregnancy and control the menstrual cycle. Thus, if you are certain that you have had all the children you want, you may feel that your ovaries are no longer required. This is a long way from the truth. The hormone oestrogen produced by the ovaries has many other functions apart from its actions on the uterine lining.

Even if the uterus is removed, the ovaries continue to produce the same amount of oestrogen for the remainder of their natural lifespan. It is sometimes stated that the ovaries fail earlier after a hysterectomy but recent research has not confirmed this.

Vaginal skin

This depends on oestrogen for its normal moisture. Lack of oestrogen may result in dryness, lack of lubrication and soreness during sexual intercourse. Even if you are not sexually active, vaginal dryness may become problematic. Some women find that removal of the ovaries reduces their sex drive.

Bones and blood vessels

These are partly dependent on oestrogen for optimum health. Loss of oestrogen at the time of the menopause causes gradual loss of calcium and mineral from the bones, resulting in thinning and eventually an increased risk of fractures. This condition of thin, brittle bones which often affects elderly women is known as osteoporosis. If your ovaries are removed before the natural menopause, bone loss occurs from an earlier age so there is a greater risk that you will eventually develop osteoporosis. Oestrogen also has a protective effect on blood vessels, particularly those of the heart. Women who lose their ovaries at a young age have a greater risk of heart attacks in later life.

Symptoms of the menopause

Symptoms such as hot flushes, night sweats and occasionally mood disturbances may start abruptly after removal of the ovaries. These symptoms vary in severity from woman to woman; some scarcely notice them whereas others are severely troubled for months or even years. However, onset of these symptoms can be prevented by the use of hormone replacement therapy (see below).

HORMONE REPLACEMENT THERAPY (HRT)

Loss of the ovaries need not be as drastic as implied in the previous section. If your ovaries have been removed, oestrogen can be prescribed by your doctor in the form of hormone replacement therapy

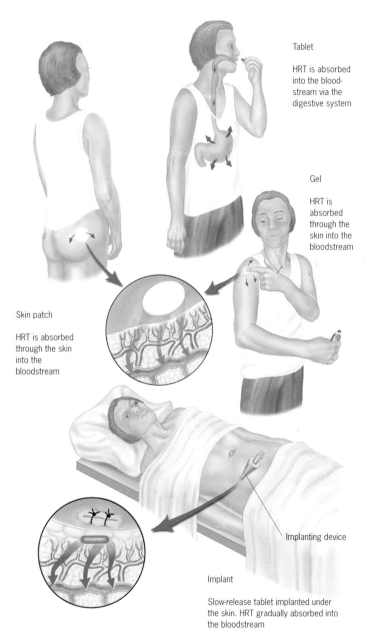

Tablet

HRT is absorbed into the bloodstream via the digestive system

Gel

HRT is absorbed through the skin into the bloodstream

Skin patch

HRT is absorbed through the skin into the bloodstream

Implanting device

Implant

Slow-release tablet implanted under the skin. HRT gradually absorbed into the bloodstream

HRT can be administered in many different ways.

(HRT). The object of this is to replace the oestrogen that is lacking and so prevent the development of the problems described above. HRT can be taken in the form of tablets, skin patches or skin gel. It is sometimes given as an implant (a small pellet inserted under the skin), although there are disadvantages to this method and some doctors do not use it. Unlike women prescribed HRT who still have a uterus, women who have had a hysterectomy need only one of the two hormones normally produced by the ovaries (oestrogen but not progesterone). HRT suits most women although for some it takes a certain amount of trial and error before they find a preparation that suits them. A minority of women find it impossible to take HRT.

Is HRT suitable for everyone?

As HRT is designed to replace hormones normally produced by the ovaries, it is suitable for most women. However, if you have had treatment for breast cancer or are having a hysterectomy for uterine lining cancer (endometrial cancer), it is not advisable to take HRT. It is also not suitable for women with a strong history of thrombosis (blood clots). There are some medical conditions for which additional health checks are required if HRT is taken. The most common of these is high blood pressure. However, as HRT has to be prescribed by a doctor, you will be asked a series of questions about your health before HRT is prescribed and this will give an opportunity to raise any concerns that you may have.

Does HRT have any side effects?

Side effects may occur with HRT but most of these are similar to the symptoms that women often experience along with their monthly cycle. The most common are sore breasts, headaches, bloating and fluid retention, but it is unlikely that you would experience all of these. Side effects can often be relieved by prescribing a lower dose of HRT or trying a different preparation. HRT may cause bleeding problems but this is not relevant if you are taking HRT after a hysterectomy. The main concern raised by women starting HRT is whether they will gain weight. Again this varies and HRT can certainly aggravate an existing weight problem. Any initial weight gain is temporary when you first start HRT and does not usually continue.

Women are naturally concerned about potential risks with HRT. On balance, it is felt that the health benefits of HRT outweigh any risks. Not only does HRT treat menopausal symptoms such as sweats and vaginal dryness, and improves the way that you feel, it also protects against bone loss and heart disease. However, the latter protective effects are only present if you take HRT for several years and not all women want or need to take HRT long term. The disadvantage of long-term HRT is that there is an increased risk of breast cancer if HRT is taken for more than five years. This risk does not apply if HRT is taken for less than five years.

All women are individuals and have different concerns and health factors. It is helpful to discuss the subject with a doctor who is interested in the menopause. For more information readers are referred to the companion booklet in this series, *Understanding the Menopause & HRT*.

Ovarian disease

If your ovaries are diseased, you are better off without them and this may be the major reason for the hysterectomy operation. For example, if you have severe endometriosis (see page 11) or if ovarian cancer is suspected, the best treatment is removal of the uterus and both ovaries. The other main reason why gynaecologists recommend removal of the ovaries is to prevent the later development of ovarian cancer. This is a very serious condition that is hard to treat, although it is not common. Some women are at increased risk of developing

ovarian cancer because they have a strong family history of this condition. Although removal of both ovaries is the best way of preventing ovarian cancer, it does not give an absolute guarantee because some ovarian cells may be left behind. Women who have no children, who have never been on the oral contraceptive pill and who have a history of infertility are at slightly greater risk. However, in general it is almost impossible to predict which women will develop ovarian cancer in the future and it can be argued that removal of healthy ovaries is an unnecessary interference with nature.

Removal of healthy ovaries

If the reason for your hysterectomy is heavy menstrual bleeding and your ovaries are healthy, removing them is not a necessary part of your treatment. Few gynaecologists would suggest doing so if you are under the age of 45 because it is generally believed that the disadvantages outweigh the advantages. If you are already menopausal or very near the menopause, it may be suggested that you should have your ovaries removed, even if they are healthy, on the basis that they are no longer functioning adequately. However, the decline in hormone production in the lead-up to and after the natural menopause is much more gradual than the sudden fall that occurs after surgical removal of the ovaries. If you request removal of your ovaries you should be well informed about HRT and feel happy about taking it.

If you suffer from severe PMS or PMT, removal of both your ovaries may be recommended on the basis that the symptoms are triggered by the hormonal changes of the menstrual cycle. However, this is a particularly drastic approach to the problem and does not always work in any case. Even worse, you may then find that HRT does not suit you. By giving a course of medical treatment that stops the production of hormones from the ovaries (a GnRH agonist – see page 28) and then later adding in some HRT, it should be possible to predict which women may benefit from removal of the ovaries.

When should HRT be started?

After a hysterectomy with removal of the ovaries, the symptoms of sudden hormone loss may start almost immediately, although they may be masked by other changes related to the operation. Feelings of being very hot and sweaty may be confused with symptoms of a fever and changes in mood with the stress of surgery. Hormone lack may contribute to feelings of anxiety and low mood after the operation, and thus there are advantages in starting HRT very early in order to

prevent these symptoms, although this should not be before you are fully mobile – usually around the time that you are due to be discharged home. The HRT may be supplied by the hospital or you can arrange for your GP to do this.

There may be medical reasons for delaying the start of HRT or you may wish to wait and see whether you really need it. Not everyone experiences symptoms after removal of their ovaries and the symptoms may be milder if you are already going through the menopause anyway. However, if you are under 45 or have additional risk factors for developing osteoporosis or heart disease in later life, HRT is strongly recommended. If you are not sure whether you are at additional risk of developing health problems later on or wish to discuss HRT in more detail, ask your GP for advice and look out for leaflets which are available in surgeries and hospital clinics. The staff of Well Woman Clinics are always willing to advise or there may be a specialised menopause clinic in your area.

What type of HRT should you be taking?

As indicated above, HRT can be taken in various ways and consists of the two hormones oestrogen and progesterone. Taking oestrogen relieves the side effects of the menopause whereas progesterone is necessary for women who still have a uterus, in order to balance out the effects of oestrogen which, on its own, could lead to abnormal thickening of the lining, bleeding problems and possibly a risk of cancer. You will need to take progesterone if you have had endometrial ablation because some remnants of the uterine lining usually remain, but it is not required after a hysterectomy. The only exception is that some women who have had a hysterectomy with removal of their ovaries for severe endometriosis require progesterone along with oestrogen to ensure that there is no reactivation of any endometriotic tissue still remaining.

The most common way of taking oestrogen is by tablet or skin patch. With tablets the hormones are absorbed through the stomach; with patches they are absorbed directly into the bloodstream through the skin. Most preparations have at least two dose strengths. Some doctors always start off by prescribing a lower dose, increasing it if the symptoms are not relieved, whereas others may base their decision on your age, using a higher dose if you are below a certain age. There is no magic formula and it may involve a degree of trial and error. Similarly, patches and tablets are equally effective and your personal preference is the most

important factor. The best way is to start with one preparation. Your doctor can then make any necessary changes based on how well your symptoms are relieved and whether you experience any side effects. Some gynaecologists will offer to insert an implant of oestrogen at the time of the operation. This goes just under the skin of the lower abdomen or buttock and lasts for about six months. Further implants are then inserted at the hospital clinic and you will need regular blood tests to measure oestrogen levels because this method can sometimes cause oestrogen levels to be too high. For this reason, implants are less commonly used than the other methods. You'll find more information about HRT in the companion booklet in this series *(Understanding Menopause & HRT)*.

Hysterectomy and your menopause

The term 'menopause' is used to describe natural failure of the ovaries and you know it has happened when your periods stop. For those who no longer have a uterus, this change is rather meaningless because you are no longer having periods, so there is no easily recognised sign that your ovaries have stopped functioning. It used to be said that ovaries fail earlier after a hysterectomy but this has been disproved by recent research.

You will most probably become aware that you are going through the menopause because you start to experience symptoms such as hot flushes or night sweats. If you are in any doubt, it can be confirmed by measurement of hormone levels in your blood. You can then discuss the need for HRT with your doctor.

KEY POINTS

✓ Removal of the ovaries is not an automatic part of a hysterectomy and may have serious implications for future health

✓ The hormone oestrogen, produced by the ovaries, has an important function in preserving the health of the vagina, bones and blood vessels

✓ Recent research has shown that, if ovaries are left behind, they do not fail any sooner after a hysterectomy

✓ If the ovaries have to be removed, hormone replacement therapy (HRT) is suitable for most women

✓ HRT can be taken as tablets, skin patches or implants under the skin

Possible complications

Most women would welcome the prospect of being free of periods for ever: the sense of freedom, no need to carry protection, no feeling of anticipation each month. This is especially so if menstruation has been a time of particular misery or anxiety with severe discomfort, flooding, prolonged bleeding or chronic anaemia. However, removal of the uterus leads to permanent loss of fertility, and involves the risks of major surgery and, if the ovaries are removed as well, sudden onset of the menopause. It is not something to be embarked upon lightly or for relatively trivial reasons. The purpose of this chapter is to describe some of the problems that might arise during or after the operation. Most of them are relatively minor and easily treatable. While you're reading this section, please do bear in mind that serious complications are rare.

THE OPERATION

Any type of operation involves risks, the most common being haemorrhage (blood loss). If this should happen, you may need a blood transfusion, depending on the severity of the bleeding. Damage to the bladder or bowel, the structures that lie beside the uterus, is very uncommon but potentially serious. Damage to the bladder is more common in women who have previously had a caesarean section because the bladder can stick to the lower part of the uterus and the cervix. For this reason, you may be advised to opt for a subtotal hysterectomy (see page 31) if you've had a number of caesarean sections. However, repair of bladder injuries is usually straightforward and the bladder works normally afterwards. More seriously, the ureters which carry urine from the kidneys to the bladder may be damaged during hysterectomy. This is very uncommon and usually occurs only in complicated cases, for example, in women with very large fibroids or those who have had previous pelvic operations. Operations for severe endometriosis are more difficult if the disease has resulted in the bowel becoming stuck to the back of the uterus, because this may increase the risk of damage to the bowel during the operation.

The gynaecologists carrying out these operations take every precaution to minimise risk, blood is always available for transfusion if necessary, and antibiotics are used to prevent and treat infection. Damage to other structures is extremely rare, occurring in about two per cent of hysterectomies, but if it does occur it may complicate and prolong the recovery time and further surgery may be required.

The anaesthetic may pose risks, particularly if you have other health problems such as heart or lung disease or are a heavy smoker. Risks are greater with general anaesthetics and can be reduced with the use of spinal or epidural anaesthetics but the latter are not suitable for everyone.

COMMON COMPLICATIONS

Problems are common during the recovery time, but most are minor and easily treated.

- Wound infections are most likely to affect women who are overweight and, although rarely serious, they may considerably delay recovery.

- Chest infections are common in smokers and those with a history of chest problems.

- Urinary infections are the most common infections overall because many women encounter difficulty in passing urine immediately after surgery. For this reason, a fine plastic tube called a catheter is left in the bladder to drain the urine during the first 24 hours after the operation, but this in turn may make a urinary infection more likely.

- Bowel upsets, such as constipation and flatulence, affect nearly everyone, but are only temporary.

- Pain and stiffness from the operation itself are almost universal, although moving around helps. Although rest is important to help the healing process, you should never lie in bed for a long time after an operation. The nurses will help you gradually to regain mobility after the operation and the physiotherapist will advise you about suitable exercises.

- Anaemia may be a problem for some women after a hysterectomy, as a result of blood loss. This can aggravate feelings of tiredness and lethargy but is quickly put right with iron tablets, although severe anaemia, causing weakness, dizziness and lightheadedness, is best corrected by a blood transfusion.

Pelvic infection

Pelvic infections, at the operation site deep down in the pelvis, affect around five per cent of women. This may be because there has been some postoperative bleeding leading to a so-called haematoma (collection of blood) which then becomes infected. The condition is diagnosed because recovery is slower than usual, and the woman has a high temperature and anaemia. The doctor may be able to feel the presence of a haematoma when doing a pelvic examination or see it on an ultrasound scan. Treatment is with antibiotics. The haematoma either heals gradually or drains through the scar at the top of the vagina; it gives rise to a temporary but very unpleasant and heavy discharge which brings rapid relief of the problem.

Occasionally there may be fresh vaginal bleeding several days after the operation. This may also be a sign of infection and should be treated promptly with antibiotics. It must not be confused with the normal discharge of some old blood or the pinkish discharge that commonly occurs as the stitches at the top of the vagina start to dissolve.

Venous thrombosis

More serious is the risk of blood clots in the deep veins of the legs or pelvis (deep venous thrombosis or DVT). If it isn't spotted quickly, clots may pass to the lungs (pulmonary embolism) which is life threatening. Hospital staff are very aware of this potential risk, hence the use of inflatable boots to maintain the circulation through your legs during the operation (you will probably not be aware of these) and of elastic support stockings when you're back on the ward. It helps to move around and do plenty of leg exercises, especially in the early stages after the operation. If you are at particular risk of blood clots or if you have had one in the past, you will be prescribed heparin injections (which reduce the blood's tendency to clot) as an extra precaution.

Additional risk factors

If you are overweight or a heavy smoker, you are at greater risk of developing problems during or after surgery. Smokers are more prone to chest infections and, as smoking is now forbidden in most hospitals, it really is worth making a huge effort to cut down on your smoking before any operation. Hysterectomy is rarely advised for women who are seriously over-weight because of the greater risk of wound and pelvic infections, venous thrombosis, anaesthetic difficulties and, in the case of prolapse, recurrence of the problem.

Longer-term consequences

Most women feel much better after a hysterectomy once they have recovered from the actual operation, but a few have serious regrets, usually because they had reservations beforehand or had not fully thought through the consequences. It is important that women who have lost their ovaries are given adequate hormone replacement to relieve or prevent menopausal symptoms.

Loss of fertility

Changes in family circumstances affect many more people today than in earlier generations, and a young woman who has had a hysterectomy may come to regret it later on if she meets a new partner. On the other hand, some gynaecological problems that reduce fertility such as endometriosis or large uterine fibroids are also cured by hysterectomy, and this can lead to bitterly difficult decisions for some women. Loss of the uterus means permanent loss of the ability to bear a child but for some women this can be a positive decision if it has been preceded by years of suffering.

Your sex life

Most women encounter no difficulty with their sex lives once they have fully recovered from a hysterectomy. Indeed many say things actually get better on that front, although a minority feel that their orgasms are less intense following the removal of the cervix. Very occasionally, a woman may feel the loss of her fertility as a psychological blow which has a negative effect on her sex drive but this reaction is not common. Removal of the ovaries is likely to give rise to problems such as vaginal dryness and painful intercourse but this is treatable with hormones (see page 51). It can also be helped by the use of lubricants such as KY jelly. A minority of women find that removal of their ovaries causes loss of sex drive that is not relieved by standard forms of HRT.

Urinary function

The urinary bladder which stores and empties urine lies very close to the uterus and urinary problems are very common after a hysterectomy. These include urinary infections, inability to pass urine and the need to pass urine more frequently or more urgently. Such difficulties are usually only temporary but a minority of women experience more persistent problems. If you had any bladder problems before your operation, you're more likely to experience them afterwards as well.

Bowel function

Constipation is extremely common in people of all ages, including women who have had hysterectomies. Few women develop constipation for the first time after hysterectomy but the operation may aggravate an already existing problem. It may take many weeks for the bowels to recover fully after a hysterectomy, but there is no evidence that any permanent changes occur.

Psychological factors

Hysterectomy will relieve your period problems, but it will not change your personality or your family circumstances, for better or worse! There is no evidence that women undergoing hysterectomy become depressed although removal of the ovaries, if untreated by HRT, may cause some unpleasant symptoms. If you have had unrealistic expectations about hysterectomy you may feel disappointed with the results afterwards, and some women will experience a reaction to loss of fertility. You are less likely to have any negative reactions if your decision to go ahead with a hysterectomy was properly thought out and discussed beforehand.

KEY POINTS

✓ Hysterectomy leads to permanent loss of fertility and involves the risks of major surgery

✓ Minor complications, such as chest, wound and pelvic infections, are common but easily treated

✓ Serious complications are rare but may considerably prolong recovery time and necessitate further surgery

✓ Complications are more common in women who smoke heavily, are overweight or have other health problems

✓ Temporary upsets in mood and in bowel and bladder function occur commonly but these return to normal during the recovery period

Preparation for a hysterectomy

Usually you will arrive at a decision about whether to have a hysterectomy gradually and after you've tried various medical treatments. This may have involved several appointments at a hospital clinic as well as visits to your GP. More rarely, the decision has to be made quickly with little time for adequate consideration. Many women welcome the operation; others view it with fear and dismay. It is only natural to feel apprehensive. Having a major operation does not affect only you as an individual, it also has an impact on your partner, your family and your employer. The better informed and prepared you all are beforehand, the less anxious you will be and the inconvenience can then be kept to a minimum for all concerned.

WHAT HAPPENS AT THE CLINIC?

The decision in favour of hysterectomy is usually made jointly and involves not only yourself but also your partner, your GP and the hospital gynaecologist. Above all, you must feel that this is the best solution for your particular problem and that you will have no regrets afterwards. Depending on the nature of the problem, this will usually mean that you have given medical therapies a fair try. You should have been made aware of any other medical or surgical alternatives and had adequate time to give these further consideration. As discussed on page 30, there are several different types of hysterectomy and it is important to understand what type of operation is proposed and for what reason. In addition, it is very important for you to know whether the gynaecologist recommends removal of the ovaries.

You should leave the hospital clinic feeling that you have been adequately informed or, if not, that you have been given someone to contact within the hospital for more information or access to reading material. You should be told how long you can expect to wait for the operation and about the arrangements that will be made regarding admission. You need to find out roughly how long you will be in hospital and how long it will be before you are fully recovered from the operation, so that you can prepare your family and employer well in advance.

HOW LONG WILL YOU BE IN HOSPITAL?

A book like this one can give only general advice, so it is important to find out as much as possible from your own hospital because things are done differently in different places. Do not rely too much on what friends and relatives may tell you; hospital practices have changed enormously and it is now quite normal for a woman to leave hospital three or four days after an abdominal hysterectomy whereas, even five years ago, she would have been kept in for seven or even ten days! This is not purely because of bed shortages but because doctors, nurses and physiotherapists have found that you will recover more easily if you are encouraged to return to normal activities more quickly. Remember that it was not all that long ago that women were made to stay in bed for a week after normal childbirth.

The hospital stay will be shorter if you are having a vaginal or laparoscopically assisted hysterectomy. It will be longer if there are any complications or if you have any additional health problems. Also, if the hysterectomy is being done for cancer, the operation itself and the recovery process may be more complicated. The hospital staff need to be made aware of your home circumstances, for example, if you live alone or have a dependent elderly relative or very young children. However, as far as possible you will be expected to make your own arrangements for additional help where necessary. Where circumstances are particularly difficult, your GP or the social services department may be able to offer advice.

GETTING BACK TO WORK

How long this takes differs enormously from person to person and also depends on the type of work you do and the operation itself. It is usual to recommend a minimum of six weeks off work. Some women who have had vaginal or laparoscopically assisted hysterectomies may be ready to return to work earlier, although after an abdominal hysterectomy it may take up to 12 weeks to recover fully. Recovery is discussed more fully on page 72. Once you are discharged from hospital, your GP is responsible for issuing 'sick lines' for your employer and will therefore keep in touch with your progress.

GETTING READY FOR THE OPERATION

If you are in good health, there are no special preparations to be made before surgery but try not to overdo it! Many women tire themselves out doing a lot extra, at home or at work, before coming in to hospital and this has an impact on how easily they recover afterwards.

If you are overweight, you may have been advised to lose weight before the operation. This is sensible advice because not only is the surgery more difficult if you are overweight, but there is also a greater risk of complications – both from the operation itself and from the anaesthetic. You should also try hard to cut down on smoking (or preferably give up altogether) to reduce your risk of a chest infection after the operation. A smoker's cough makes your wound more painful and puts more strain on the stitch line and on your pelvic floor. Remember that many hospitals operate a no-smoking policy so you won't be allowed to smoke during your hospital stay.

If you suffer from health problems, such as asthma, diabetes or high blood pressure, it is important that the hospital doctors know what medications you normally take so that any necessary adjustments can be made during and immediately after the operation. Most treatments that you are taking already should continue but, if in any doubt, do ask the hospital staff.

ADMISSION ARRANGEMENTS

In some hospitals women are admitted to hospital on the day before the operation; others have a pre-admission clinic that you attend a week or so in advance and then you are admitted on the day of the operation. Either way, the purpose is to complete a certain amount of paper work relevant to your admission, carry out a routine health check and ensure that you are fully informed about the nature of your operation. Routine investigations may include a chest X-ray, ECG (to check for any abnormality of your heart beat) and blood tests. This will include blood for cross-matching (in case you require a blood transfusion during or after the operation). You will be given a Consent Form to read through and sign. This gives the gynaecologist permission to carry out the operation and you must be sure that you understand the nature of the operation and what you are consenting to. This is an opportunity to ask questions and to seek further clarification about any issues of uncertainty, for example, whether or not your ovaries will be removed.

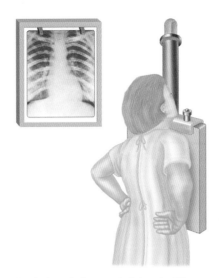

Routine investigations may include a chest X-ray.

THE ANAESTHETIC

Hysterectomy may be carried out under a general or a regional (local) anaesthetic which is usually combined with a sedative or light general anaesthetic as well. The anaesthetist will visit you before the operation to discuss the anaesthetic, check up on your general health and find out what medication you may be taking. He or she will explain what will happen and will want

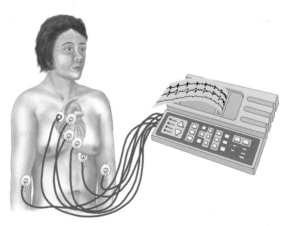

An ECG will confirm that your heart is working normally.

to know if you have any particular concerns. You may be offered a 'pre-med' to help you relax which may make you drowsy. It is usually a tablet or capsule taken about an hour before you are brought along for the operation.

On the day of the operation you will not be allowed anything to eat or drink. This is to keep your stomach empty because, if you are sick while under the anaesthetic, there is a risk that you might inhale your stomach contents into your lungs. A nurse from the ward as well as a theatre nurse or orderly will go with you to the operating theatre. When you arrive for the operation, you will be connected to several routine monitors. These are to measure your pulse, blood pressure and blood oxygen level during the operation. You will have a drip put into the back of your hand or at the bend of your arm so you can be given fluids during and after the operation when you are unable to drink. It is also used to give drugs or a blood transfusion if necessary.

A general anaesthetic is given by injecting drugs into the drip that will send you off to sleep. Before this you may be given oxygen to breathe through a mask. Once you are asleep, the anaesthetic is usually continued with anaesthetic gases. The anaesthetist will stay with you, charting your progress during the operation. Muscle relaxa-

tion is necessary for an operation to be done, so a muscle relaxant drug is given. Your breathing is taken over by a ventilator, connected to your lungs by a tube placed in the windpipe. During the operation, you'll receive pain-killing drugs to reduce your bodily reactions to the surgery and to ensure that, when you wake up, the pain is under control. At the end of the operation, a drug is given to reverse the effect of the muscle relaxant. The anaesthetic gases are stopped and oxygen is given.

A regional anaesthetic will either be a spinal anaesthetic (a single injection into the spinal canal) or an epidural (when a fine tube is inserted into the epidural space around the spinal canal). To place these, the anaesthetist will ask you to bend your back so that the injection can be made easily. Once the effects of the anaesthetic have been checked, it is usual to give a sedative or a light general anaesthetic so that you know very little about what goes on during the operation. Regional anaesthetics block nerves to and from the lower part of your body so you won't be able to feel anything or even move your legs for a while. A regional anaesthetic may be preferable to a general anaesthetic for people with heart or chest problems. It may also help with pain relief after the operation.

WAKING UP

You will wake up in the recovery area. The nurses and the anaesthetist will check to make sure that you are breathing well and that you have had enough pain-killers. Oxygen treatment will continue for some time after the operation because anaesthetics and pain-killers tend to reduce the normal blood oxygen levels. The catheter placed in your bladder during the operation to keep it empty may be left in afterwards in case you have difficulty passing urine yourself. It is connected through the tube into a bag at the side of the bed. Measuring the amount of urine in the bag is a good way of checking that things are going well after the operation. A drain may be left in the wound, either through the abdomen or, in the case of a vaginal hysterectomy, through the vagina, so any blood loss after the operation can be measured and to prevent it collecting in the pelvis. Antibiotics are usually given just before or during the operation to reduce the risk of infection. Some people are allergic to certain antibiotics so it is most important that you tell the doctor beforehand of any allergies that you have to any medication.

VISITORS

You need to find out your hospital's policy regarding visitors in advance,

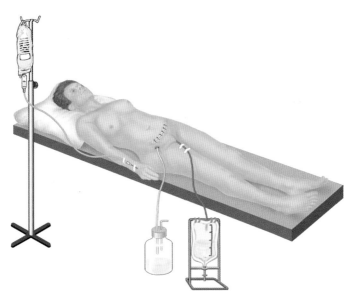

After your operation you will wake up in the recovery area.

but only very close relatives are likely to be allowed in on the day of the operation because you will be very sleepy. Thereafter visitors are welcome but too many at one time is tiring for yourself and for your fellow patients. Staff are always willing to answer your relatives' questions and keep them in touch with your progress, although information given out over the phone is usually limited because it is not possible to verify the identity of callers. Pay phones are available on all wards but the use of mobile phones is usually forbidden because of possible interference with medical monitoring equipment.

KEY POINTS

✓ Medical treatments should be given a fair try and other surgical options considered before deciding on a hysterectomy

✓ Hysterectomies may be carried out under a general or regional (spinal or epidural) anaesthetic

✓ Preparation for hysterectomy includes a detailed explanation of the procedures to be undertaken and a general health check, including blood tests

✓ The consent form gives the gynaecologist permission to carry out the operation and women must be certain about the details of what they are signing

✓ It is important that the hospital staff, especially the anaesthetist, are fully informed about any health problems, medications and allergies

After the operation

THE FIRST 24 HOURS

Recovering from an operation is a different experience for everyone. At least you can feel relief that it is all over. Initially you will most probably have a drip in your arm, a catheter in your bladder and possibly a wound drain. If you had an epidural anaesthetic, the epidural tube may still be in place in your back. All these tubes will gradually be removed as your recovery progresses and you become more mobile.

Pain relief

Pain relief depends on what type of operation you had; an abdominal hysterectomy involves an incision that is more painful than a vaginal hysterectomy. Initially you are given pain-killers such as morphine (known as opiates) which don't suppress the pain completely but make it bearable and help you to relax. Once your pain is under control, you may be allowed to give yourself small extra doses whenever you need to by pressing a button on a small machine that controls the flow of pain-killing drug through the drip in your arm. The machine 'locks out' for a time after each dose so there is no risk of you taking too much. Additional pain-killers may be given if required.

You must try to move around too, even though it hurts, because this helps to prevent complications such as blood clots or chest infections. Try to take an occasional deep breath and cough if you feel like it. If you have had a spinal or epidural anaesthetic you will have no pain until the anaesthetic wears off. You will have to tell the nurses as soon as you feel any discomfort as the pain may build up quite quickly. With epidurals, the local anaesthetic effect can be kept going if an epidural catheter was placed in your back, so that anaesthetics or pain-killers can be injected later when you need them. When you no longer need powerful pain-killers and are able to move around, you'll be given milder and less frequent pain-killers instead. Taking these regularly is more effective than waiting until the pain gets too bad.

Nausea and vomiting can be a problem, particularly if you are prone to travel sickness or have had the same problem with previous anaesthetics. Modern treatments are much better than older drugs so sickness should not be a big problem for most people.

THE NEXT 24 TO 48 HOURS

You are not usually allowed to drink or eat on the day of the operation. You should be able to drink fluids on the day after the operation and to eat by the second day. Following surgery, the bowel tends to become rather sluggish, and this can cause nausea, flatulence and constipation. Painful passage of wind plagues many women after hysterectomy but fortunately this is a very temporary problem. Passing urine may feel strange initially and this is normal, but you should let the nurse know if it feels sore or if you have a frequent urge to pass small amounts of urine as this may be a symptom of a urinary tract infection.

On the first day after the operation you will be bed-bathed and allowed up to sit in a chair. You will be taken to the bathroom for a shower on your second day. If you have had a vaginal or laparoscopically assisted hysterectomy, you will be able to get up sooner. Movement is important after an operation because it helps to relieve pain and stiffness and also helps to prevent deep vein thrombosis (blood clots in the legs). As there is a risk of this after a hysterectomy, you may have to wear strong supporting tights or stockings, and some women are given injections of an anti-clotting drug called heparin if they are felt to be at extra risk of thrombosis.

At this stage, you will still require pain-killers and you should ask for them in good time, before the pain gets too bad.

The staff team

A team of nursing staff will look after you during your stay in the ward, liaise with your relatives and help you to plan your discharge home. One of the team is your 'named nurse' who has particular responsibility for your care. Take every opportunity to ask questions; the staff are there to help. There is also a team of doctors, headed by a consultant, and one of them will visit you every day to assess your progress and answer any questions that you might have. The gynaecologist who performed your operation will give you information about the operation itself. Make sure that you are clear about whether you still have your ovaries and, if not, whether and when you should start hormone replacement therapy if you haven't done so already. The physiotherapist will come and give you advice about mobility and a routine of gentle exercises which you should do regularly to assist your recovery.

The pathology report

The uterus and any other organs that have been removed are examined by a pathologist as a matter of routine and the report is filed in your case notes. Unless an urgent report is requested, it takes seven to 10 days for it to be completed, by which time you will have gone home. However, your GP is usually informed of the result in the discharge letter that is routinely sent out, summarising your hospital stay. If you want to know the results as soon as possible, you can arrange to contact a member of the hospital staff at the appropriate time.

GOING HOME

Minor complications are common after hysterectomy (see page 73). Most are easily treated and should not unduly prolong your stay in hospital. Most hospitals have a very flexible policy about when you can go home. If you have good home support you will be allowed home as soon as you feel well enough. After a laparoscopically assisted or vaginal hysterectomy this may be as early as the second or third post-operative day, but is more likely to be between three and six days after an abdominal hysterectomy. If there are abdominal sutures or staples to be removed, arrangements can be made for this to be done as an outpatient or by the district nurse. Often dissolving sutures are used which do not require removal.

The early recovery period

It is usual to feel very tired and rather 'low' in the early days and even weeks; an operation is very stressful both physically and emotionally and you will need plenty of rest. You probably won't feel up to anything more than light reading, sewing and watching television, and you should avoid taking on household or family responsibilities until you feel able to cope. There may also be times during the recovery period when you feel rather depressed or emotional, which is a perfectly natural reaction that will pass.

Return to normal activities

When it comes to physical activities, take it slowly, but you should be able to bath, shower, walk up and down stairs, and make drinks and light snacks by the end of the first week. Make a real effort to do the exercises prescribed by the physiotherapist on a regular basis. By the second or third week you can go out for short walks, go shopping (but don't carry heavy bags or push a trolley) and make light meals. You can start to swim and drive by the fourth or fifth week and do light housework. Within six to eight weeks you should be getting back to all your normal activities, including work and sport. You can start to resume your sex life if you feel ready but take it slowly. Your partner is likely to feel equally apprehensive! It is better not to have full penetrative sex until you have had an internal examination which is usually carried out at the hospital or by your GP six weeks after the operation. The purpose of this is to make sure that the scar at the top of the vagina has healed properly. Occasionally healing may not be complete and so-called 'granulation tissue' may have formed. This can cause bleeding and discomfort on intercourse but can be easily treated so do tell your doctor if it happens.

COMMON PROBLEMS

Problems can arise after discharge from hospital. It is usual to feel some pain and discomfort and you should have been prescribed some pain-killers, which you'll probably need to take for up to two weeks

after the operation. Your pain should gradually lessen during this time but there will be times when you are aware of it, for example, when you are tired or have been more active than before. If your pain worsens for no obvious reason and you feel unwell and develop a fever, you should contact your doctor as this may be a sign of infection.

Passing urine may not feel entirely normal and if you have any symptoms suggestive of an infection, such as burning and a desire to pass urine very frequently, you should drink plenty of fluids and arrange through your GP to have a sample of urine tested. Bowel problems are extremely common and are in part related to the operation itself and also to the upset in your normal diet and routine. They will gradually settle as you return to normal. An abdominal scar may cause problems such as discomfort, lumpiness, bruising and slight stickiness or discharge. It is normal for the skin area above the scar to feel numb because some of the nerves supplying the skin were cut. Nerves are extremely slow to heal so the numbness will persist for many months. Odd skin sensations and even sharp pains around the scar are common during the healing process.

If the wound becomes very red, tender and hot, this is usually the result of a wound infection and you should contact your GP as you will need antibiotics. Minor wound discharge does not require any special attention other than a clean dressing. After a wound infection or if there has been a lot of bruising, there may be a heavy discoloured or offensive discharge from the wound and you will need help from the district or practice nurse. There is also likely to be some dark-brown discharge from the stitch line at the top of the vagina and this can last for two to three weeks. If it becomes heavy, offensive or bright red this may be a sign of infection and you should contact your doctor. It's better to use sanitary pads rather than tampons during this time, to reduce the risk of infection.

You may notice that your tummy bulges out: this is caused by temporary loss of muscle tone and will recover as you exercise. Similarly the muscles of the pelvic floor become rather slack, hence the importance of doing the regular pelvic floor and abdominal wall exercises shown to you by the physiotherapist.

Apart from the physical problems described above, some women may experience emotional symptoms, although these are usually just a short-lived reaction to the stress of the operation, and it's normal to feel tired and lethargic for some time after surgery. Emotional symptoms following removal of the ovaries and other symptoms of the menopause can be treated with HRT.

THE POSTOPERATIVE CHECK

It is normal to be seen at the hospital or by your GP at your GP's surgery about six weeks after the operation. By this point, you should be fully recovered or well on your way to full recovery and the scars should have healed. You'll have an internal examination so the doctor can inspect the scar at the top of the vagina and ensure that healing is complete. The visit will give you an opportunity to ask questions and discuss any concerns. If you had your ovaries removed and have started HRT, the doctors will want to find out whether you are experiencing any problems with it. If for some reason HRT was delayed, this will be an opportunity to discuss whether and when you should start it.

KEY POINTS

✓ Nausea, vomiting and pain are common early on, but medication will be given to relieve these problems

✓ Movement is particularly important after an operation because it helps to prevent stiffness, pain and venous thrombosis

✓ An abdominal hysterectomy involves on average three to six days in hospital, varying according to general health and individual circumstances

✓ Most women can drive a car after three to four weeks, and return to work after six to twelve weeks, depending on their speed of recovery and the nature of their work

✓ Women can expect to return to a normal sex life after a hysterectomy

Case histories

MARY

Mary G is a 43-year-old secretary who was sterilised eight years ago after the birth of her third child. Before that she had used the 'pill' for contraception before and between pregnancies. Since stopping the 'pill', her periods had become increasingly heavy and at first she could cope, but lately she'd been finding that for the first three days she had to use double or even triple protection. On one occasion her period started unexpectedly early at work and she had a very embarrassing accident which prompted a visit to her GP.

The doctor gave Mary a pelvic examination and found her uterus to be slightly bulky. Suspecting the presence of a fibroid, she organised an ultrasound scan. A blood test showed that Mary was mildly anaemic so iron tablets were prescribed. The ultrasound scan showed no obvious fibroids and the ovaries

were healthy. After discussion, her doctor prescribed Cyclokapron (tranexamic acid) tablets to reduce the amount of bleeding. She was to take two of these three or four times daily, starting once the bleeding became heavy. Mary found these quite helpful, provided that she took them four times daily for five days each month, but, if she delayed or forgot the tablets, her bleeding was again very heavy. She also found that her cycle was becoming shorter, giving her less of an interval in between her periods. This trend towards a shorter cycle had started even before she commenced the Cyclokapron and her GP confirmed that it was not a side effect of the medication. She offered Mary some hormone tablets to take during the second half of the cycle in order to delay the onset of bleeding, but Mary declined these as she felt that she was already taking enough tablets. Her sister had had a hysterectomy and she wondered if this would be an option for her too.

She was referred to a gynaecologist at the local hospital who examined her and took a biopsy from the uterine lining. They discussed the various options. The gynaecologist advised her that a vaginal hysterectomy would be possible and would result in a shorter hospital stay and recovery time than an abdominal operation. They also discussed endometrial ablation but Mary felt that she would rather have an operation that would guarantee a cure, but wanted to know whether her ovaries would be removed. The gynaecologist explained that it was not his policy to remove ovaries unless they were diseased and that the earlier scan had shown them to be healthy.

Twelve months later Mary has had no regrets about the operation, although she did feel that it took a little longer for her to recover than she had expected. This was because she was anaemic after the operation and had developed a pelvic infection, although this was successfully treated with antibiotics.

HELEN

Helen McC was 39 when she first went to her GP complaining of heavy periods. She had also been aware of some abdominal swelling but had thought that she was putting on weight because pressure of work had meant she'd stopped going to her exercise classes. After an examination, her doctor told her that she had a greatly enlarged uterus, most probably caused by fibroids. He warned her that she might need a hysterectomy, arranged an ultrasound scan to confirm the diagnosis and requested an appointment with a local gynaecologist.

Helen was somewhat dismayed at this news. She had one son, now a teenager, and had assumed she might have another child. However, she had never established a long-term relationship after the break-up of her marriage and was currently building up her career. The possible loss of her uterus was something she had not considered and she was concerned about taking time off work. She went to read up on the subject of fibroids in the library and also looked up some medical literature on the Internet.

By the time she saw the hospital consultant she was fairly well informed. The diagnosis of uterine fibroids had been confirmed and these appeared to be multiple and of various sizes, although both her ovaries were healthy. They discussed the possibility of an operation to remove only the fibroids (a myomectomy) but she understood that there would be a chance of subsequent growth of more fibroids.

Also she had already decided that further child bearing was no longer an issue for her in view of her age and current circumstances, and thus that she would prefer to have a hysterectomy which would guarantee relief from her heavy periods. Unfortunately, her consultant explained that her uterus was too large to be safely removed using keyhole surgery as she had hoped, even if she first had a course of drug injections to shrink the fibroids.

After further consideration Helen decided to go ahead with an abdominal hysterectomy. She was told that she should keep her ovaries unless she had strong views to the contrary. She requested a total hysterectomy so that she wouldn't have to bother with any more cervical smears but agreed that her cervix should be left behind if its removal was going to cause any difficulties at the time of the operation. She preferred to keep her ovaries as she did not want to have to remember to take pills or patches for the next 10 to 15 years. Despite the very large fibroids, the operation went well and she was allowed home after only four days in hospital because her mother was able to stay with her. Although very tired initially, her recovery went better than she had expected; her only problem was constipation and it took several weeks for her bowels to return to normal.

TRICIA

Tricia H had always experienced heavy painful periods and had taken the pill on and off over the years. She wanted to go back on it when, at the age of 41, her bleeding became more troublesome but her doctor was unwilling to prescribe it as she is a smoker. The doctor examined her, took a smear which was due and prescribed mefenamic acid (Ponstan), explaining that it would ease the pain and help to reduce the amount of bleeding. Tricia found that it made little difference to the bleeding and went back to her GP several months later to see if there was anything else she could try. He reassured her that her heavy periods had not caused her to be anaemic and prescribed tranexamic acid (Cyclokapron). This time her heavy bleeding seemed to improve but her next two periods were much more painful than normal. Her GP suggested that she could take mefenamic acid and tranexamic acid together, but she felt unhappy about this and stopped the tablets altogether. The next time she visited the surgery she was referred to the gynaecological clinic at the local hospital for further advice.

Examination by the gynaecologist confirmed that there was no apparent abnormality and he told her he would normally suggest she try medical treatment or endometrial ablation before considering hysterectomy. However, he also told her that the hospital was currently involved in a research study to compare the effectiveness of endometrial ablation with that of the new intrauterine device that reduces menstrual bleeding. If she agreed to take part in the study she would not choose the method of treatment, it would be chosen for her at random. She was given an information leaflet about the study and an appointment to attend an interview with the research sister. Having read the leaflet, she felt quite enthusiastic about the study and agreed to take part. She was allocated to have endometrial ablation and was prescribed an injection to thin out the uterine lining before the operation. Her next period was very much lighter as a consequence of the injection.

The operation was done in the day surgery unit. She had been warned that if there were any complications she may need to undergo additional surgery, which would involve a longer hospital stay. The operation was straightforward although she did feel unwell afterwards and spent two days in bed at home. She bled for about two weeks and this was followed by a brownish discharge which lasted for a week. As part of the study she kept a menstrual diary and was seen by the research sister at the hospital. Her first two periods after the operation failed to arrive but they did return thereafter. Twelve months after the operation there is a definite improvement in the amount of bleeding but little reduction in pain although this is relieved by pain-killers.

Questions & answers

● Will I put weight on after a hysterectomy?

Weight is not gained as a result of having a hysterectomy, but you may put on a few pounds as a consequence of being less active during the recovery period. Also it is common to have a sensation of abdominal fullness after an abdominal operation, because of the loss of tone in the abdominal muscles in the early weeks. The best plan is to take regular gentle exercise (see page 72) and to eat sensibly with plenty of fresh fruit and vegetables. You should avoid fatty foods and too much carbohydrate during the time that you are less active. Sensible eating will also help your bowels to recover a regular pattern (see page 73).

● Will having a hysterectomy affect my sex life?

The vast majority of women who have had a hysterectomy resume a normal sex life afterwards and, for some, it is improved because of the absence of worry about bleeding problems and other menstrual discomforts. There is no evidence that loss of the uterus reduces sexual arousal or enjoyment. On the other hand, a hysterectomy cannot be expected to cure sexual problems and it is most important that you discuss any difficulties and concerns beforehand with your GP or gynaecologist.

● When can I start having sex again after a hysterectomy?

It is best to delay full intercourse for six weeks after a hysterectomy and preferably until after you have had your 'six-week check-up' (see page 73), when you will be examined to ensure that the top of your vagina has fully healed. Don't worry if it takes a while for your sexual feelings to return; this is common after any operation and will improve with time as you regain your energy. If you have had your ovaries removed, you may experience dryness of the vagina and pain on intercourse. This is relieved by hormone replacement therapy (HRT). There are also non-hormonal remedies available to help with vaginal lubrication. Your GP will be able to advise you about suitable treatment.

● When can I start to drive?
This varies from woman to woman and it takes longer if you have had an abdominal hysterectomy, rather than a vaginal hysterectomy. The average is three to four weeks after an abdominal operation. Experiment by sitting in your car with the seat belt done up and practise moving the pedals up and down. Once you feel comfortable and are able to tackle an emergency stop, it is safe for you to take the car out yourself.

● When can I start exercising again?
This varies according to the type of hysterectomy, your general state of fitness before the operation, and how you feel in yourself. You should continue with the exercises that you have been taught in hospital, because these are designed to tone up your tummy and strengthen your pelvic floor

muscles. All activities should be started off gradually so that you can find your own pace. Walking is an excellent exercise that you can do right away and you can start swimming four or five weeks after the operation. You should be ready gradually to restart your normal sporting activities (for example, golf, aerobics) six to eight weeks after the operation. You are bound to tire more easily initially, but remember that exercise is beneficial both mentally and physically.

● What about housework?
Like all activities, you should build up gradually, taking particular care about your posture. Take plenty of rest and, where possible, sit rather than stand. During the first week you should be mostly resting, although you should be able to prepare light meals for yourself. Three to four weeks after the operation, you should be able to tackle most routine household tasks, with the exception of those involving heavy lifting or prolonged standing. Get someone to push the vacuum cleaner for the first four weeks after your operation because this puts a strain on the abdominal muscles.

● When should I return to work?
Again this depends on the type of hysterectomy, your general

health and your speed of recovery. After a vaginal or laparoscopically assisted hysterectomy, you may be fit to go back to work after four weeks, although recovery will take longer if you have also had a pelvic floor repair. After an abdominal hysterectomy, you should be ready after six to eight weeks, unless your job is particularly heavy. Activities that involve heavy lifting should be avoided for three months after a hysterectomy or pelvic repair.

● Is it true that a hysterectomy can cause depression?

This is not true. However, tiredness and weepiness are common in the early days after any operation, and this is partly the result of the physical stress of the operation and also of the discomfort and frustration caused when you can't do all the things that you want to do. Removal of the ovaries can affect your mood, but this can be treated by HRT (see page 51).

● Will I need HRT and when do I start it after the operation?

You will need HRT only if your ovaries have been removed at the time of the operation (or if you were already on it beforehand). HRT is usually started soon after the operation in order to prevent troublesome symptoms such as hot flushes or night sweats. It may be started while you are still in hospital or your GP may prescribe it for you once you have been discharged home. There is not usually any need to delay HRT for longer than a few days after the operation, unless you prefer to wait to see if symptoms develop. It is important that you have an opportunity to discuss HRT, preferably before the operation, but certainly with the hospital staff while you are on the ward. Once you have left hospital, your GP will prescribe HRT for you and advise you about any problems that you may experience. HRT is discussed in more detail on pages 51–6.

● Do I have to take HRT if I don't want to?

HRT is important if you have your ovaries removed well before the natural menopause. If you are aged under 45, it is unlikely that your ovaries will be removed if they are healthy but, if so, you will be advised to take HRT (see page 55). If you already menopausal or near the age of natural menopause, HRT is less important for you unless you develop troublesome symptoms (see page 51). However, some doctors encourage all women to take HRT if the ovaries are removed surgically before the natural menopause because of a sudden fall in hormone production. This is very different from natural menopause when hormone levels fall more gradually. You should discuss your concerns about HRT before deciding whether or not your ovaries should be removed.

● If I keep my ovaries, am I at risk of developing cancer?

Having a hysterectomy does not alter your later risk of developing ovarian cancer, compared with women who haven't had a hysterectomy. Indeed, it reduces it a little because your ovaries are inspected at the time of the operation and only left in if they are healthy. Obviously, removal of the ovaries reduces your risk of ovarian cancer. Ovarian cancer is not common, but some women are at greater risk than others, particularly if they have a family history of ovarian cancer (and sometimes other forms of cancer). Women who have had children are at less risk than those who have been infertile. If you were on the contraceptive pill for several years, this helps to reduce your future risk of ovarian cancer. You should discuss these risks in more detail with your gynaecologist.

● Can I choose to have a vaginal rather than an abdominal hysterectomy?

Not all women are suitable for vaginal hysterectomy (see page 32) and you will need to discuss this with the gynaecologist who is carrying out the operation. If you have large fibroids or endometriosis, you will be unlikely to be offered a vaginal hysterectomy. Women who have had normal childbirth are more suitable than those who have had no children or only caesarean section births. This is because childbirth results in some stretching of the upper vagina and of the ligaments that support the uterus, making a vaginal hysterectomy easier and safer. If you request removal of your ovaries, this may not be possible with a vaginal hysterectomy. However, some gynaecologists will recommend a laparoscopically assisted vaginal hysterectomy in which the ovaries are removed with the aid of the laparoscope and the remainder of the operation is done via the vagina (see page 34).

Useful information

Amarant Trust

Sycamore House
5 Sycamore Street
London EC1Y 0SB
Tel: 0171 608 3222
Clinic: 80 Lambeth Road
London SE1 7PW
Tel: 0171 401 3855
Fax: 0171 928 9134

Advice about the menopause and HRT.

British Association of Counselling (BAC)

1 Regent Place
Rugby
Warwickshire CV21 2PJ
Information: 01788 578328
Tel: 01788 550899
Fax: 01788 562189
Minicom: 01788 572838
Email: bac@bac.co.uk
Website: www.counselling.co.uk

Information about counselling services.

Family Planning Association

2–12 Pentonville Road
London N1 9FP
Tel: 020 7837 5432
Fax: 020 7837 3042
Web site: www.fpa.org.uk

Deals mainly with contraception, but a useful source of up-to-date information about other services and organisations relating to women's health.

Hysterectomy Support Network

For information about this and other related isues, contact:
Women's Health
52 Featherstone Street
London EC1Y 8RT
Helpline: 020 7251 6580
(Mon, Wed, Thur, Fri 10am–4pm)
Tel: 020 7251 6333
Fax: 020 7608 0928
Minicom: 020 7490 5489
Website: womenshealth@popfree.poptel.org.uk

Provides information about support groups.

National Endometriosis Society

50 Westminster Palace Gardens
Artillery Row
London SW1P 1RL
Helpline: 020 7222 2776
(2–5pm; 7–10pm)
Tel: 020 7222 2781
Email: n.info@compuserve.com
Website: www.endo.org.uk

Information, support and counselling for women with endometriosis

National Osteoporosis Society

PO Box 10
Radstock
Bath BA3 3YB
Helpline: 01761 472721
Tel: 01761 471771
Fax: 01761 471104
Email: info@nos.org.uk
Web site: www.nos.org.uk

Information about the menopause and HRT, particularly in relation to osteoporosis.

Women's Health Concern

For a publications list, send a stamped, self-addressed envelope to:
WHC Publications
Wellwood
North Farm Road

Tunbridge Wells
Kent TN2 3DR
Helpline: 0181 780 3007 (Message listing current advice numbers in various parts of the country)
Tel: 01892 510850

Women's Nationwide Cancer Control Campaign

Suna House
128–130 Curtain Road
London EC2A 3AR
Tel: 020 7729 4688
Fax: 020 7613 0771
Email: wnccc@dial.pipex.com

Encourages measures for the prevention and early detection of women's cancers. Provides information, including educational leaflets and posters.

Further reading

Hysterectomy and Vaginal Repair by Sally Haslett and Molly Jennings. Beaconsfield Publishers, UK. ISBN 0-906-58446-9 A simple guide to practical aspects of surgery and recovery.

The availability of books on this subject is very variable and some are currently out of print. Your best bet is to enquire at your local library or at a large bookshop. The most up-to-date source of information is the Internet, although some of the information available has not been subjected to critical appraisal and may be misleading. Most of the organisations listed above include leaflets on request or can advise about suitable reading material. The Royal College of Obstetricians and Gynaecologists publish booklets for patients on various subjects. For further information phone 020 7772 6276.

Index